# FAST FACTS

OUTHERN DERBYSHIRE ACUTE HO

NHS TRUST

LIBRARY & KNOWLEDGE SERVICE

## Urinar

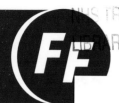

*Indispensable*
*Guides to*
*Clinical*
*Practice*

Oxford

Fast Facts – Urinary Stones
First published January 2002

Text © 2002 David A Tolley, Joseph W Segura
© 2002 in this edition Health Press Limited
Health Press Limited, Elizabeth House, Queen Street, Abingdon,
Oxford OX14 3JR, UK
Tel: +44 (0)1235 523233
Fax: +44 (0)1235 523238

Fast Facts is a trade mark of Health Press Limited.

The publisher and the authors have made every effort to ensure the
accuracy of this book, but cannot accept responsibility for any errors
or omissions.

A CIP catalogue record for this title is available from the British Library.

ISBN 1-899541-09-8

Tolley, DA (David)
Fast Facts – Urinary Stones/
David A Tolley, Joseph W Segura

Illustrated by Dee McLean, London, UK.

Printed by Fine Print (Services) Ltd, Oxford, UK.

Glossary  4

Introduction  5

Aetiology  6

Investigation and diagnosis  14

Management  19

Equipment  29

Ureteroscopy  46

Nephrostomy tubes and stents  50

Percutaneous nephrolithotomy  54

Shock-wave lithotripsy  59

Guidelines and consensus terminology  66

Future trends  74

Key references  77

Index  79

# Glossary

**Caliectasis:** ballooning of the calices associated with obstruction to the free flow of urine from the kidney or scarring

**Endoscope:** an instrument for visualization of body cavities or organs

**Fluoroscopy:** an X-ray technique used to check on progress during a procedure, such as entrapping a stone in a basket or aiming shock waves during lithotripsy

**Fr:** French or Charrière, a unit of circumference (3 Fr circumference = 1 mm diameter)

**Hydronephrosis:** distension and dilatation of the renal pelvis due to obstruction of the free flow of urine from the kidney

**IVU:** intravenous urography; radiographic visualization of the renal pelvis and ureter by injection of a radiopaque liquid into the bloodstream that is then excreted by the kidney

**Jackstone:** a combination of calcium and oxalate

**Metastable urine:** supersaturated urine without crystal formation

**Nephroscope:** an instrument to inspect the interior of the kidney

**Nephrostomy:** A surgically created passage from the skin directly into the central collecting space of the kidney. Usually a tube is left in this passage to drain urine into a bag carried outside the body. This passage can also be enlarged and used for percutaneous procedures on the kidney

**Nucleation:** crystal formation

**Parathyroidectomy:** excision of one or more parathyroid glands

**PNL:** percutaneous nephrolithotomy; removal of a stone from the kidney through an incision in the skin and via direct access into the kidney substance

**PTH:** parathyroid hormone

**Radioisotope renography:** intravenous injection of a radioactive substance that is concentrated and excreted by the kidneys. The radioisotope emits gamma rays that can be followed using a camera placed over the kidneys. The resultant data provide information on renal function and drainage

**Staghorn:** refers to the branched shape of certain (usually struvite) large stones

**Steinstrasse:** a column of stone fragments within the ureter with a large obstructing leading fragment

**Stent:** a hollow tube or mesh-like structure inserted into the ureter to maintain patency

**Struvite:** a magnesium ammonium phosphate stone produced in an alkaline environment; associated with urinary tract infection

**SWL:** shock-wave lithotripsy

**UPJ:** ureteropelvic junction

**Ureteroscope:** an instrument used to visualize the ureters and the renal collecting system

# Introduction

The management of renal and ureteric stones has evolved during the past two decades from an almost entirely surgical practice to one which is almost completely non-surgical. Indeed, open stone surgery in North America and western Europe is currently used only as a salvage procedure for certain giant staghorn stones or in other unusual situations.

This evolution has been driven by the invention of the extracorporeal shock-wave machine, the manufacture of small ureteroscopes of outstanding quality and capability, and the development of ureterorenoscopy so that all parts of the collecting system are now regularly and routinely accessible.

*Fast Facts – Urinary Stones* summarizes the state of the art in the endoscopic management of stones and the latest methods of intracorporeal stone fragmentation, and delivers a balanced perspective on the role of ureteroscopy versus shock-wave lithotripsy for the management of ureteric stones. Approaches differ between urologists in the UK, USA and continental Europe, but most of these differences are due to variation in healthcare economics rather than fundamental differences in procedure. This book is intended for house officers, junior trainees (particularly those in urology), the interested generalist, and anyone needing a quick, concise summary of the state of the art in urinary stone management.

# 1 Aetiology

The prevalence of urinary stones increased steadily throughout the twentieth century, interrupted only by the two World Wars, and is related to increased affluence and the consistent high consumption of refined carbohydrates and animal protein in the diet. Between 120 and 140 people in every 100 000 population will develop a stone each year depending on geographical location. Anyone can form a stone, but men are twice to three times as likely to form a stone as women. However, women are more likely to form an infected stone due to the increased number of urinary tract infections they suffer. People who live in certain 'stone belts', such as southeastern USA, are also more likely to form stones – the reasons for this are not known, but may be due to the presence or absence of trace elements in the soil. Overall, first-time stone formers have roughly a 10% chance per year of developing a new stone or about a 50% chance in 5 years without medical evaluation and treatment.

A surgical stone is defined as a stone that is symptomatic, causes obstruction or threatens to do so, or is a source of infection. Urinary stones can be single or multiple and vary in size and shape. They are located within the renal parenchyma or urinary collecting system. Large stones regularly cause obstruction, which can lead to hydronephrosis, kidney damage and an increased risk of infection.

Stone formation is a multifactorial and complex process. Typically, urinary stones consist of an organic protein matrix or framework that supports crystalline material composed of:
- calcium salts (73%)
- struvite (15%)
- urate (8%)
- cystine (3%)
- miscellaneous material.

Many stones are composed of combinations of crystals and miscellaneous material (Table 1.1), and it is still not possible to determine stone composition with certainty on a plain radiograph alone. Recently, computer analysis of pixel densities on computerized tomography (CT) images has

TABLE 1.1

**Type and frequency of urinary stones**

| Type of stone | Approximate frequency (%) |
|---|---|
| Calcium oxalate } Calcium phosphate | 73 |
| Struvite | 15 |
| Uric acid | 8 |
| Cystine | 3 |

been used to predict renal stone composition, but this is only possible in a non-specific way. However, if the composition of a previously passed stone is known, it is often possible to estimate the composition of a recurring stone. Typically, cystine has a ground-glass appearance, while struvite usually appears poorly calcified. Small uric acid stones are radiolucent, though large uric acid stones are faintly calcified. All types of stone occur more commonly in men than women, except for struvite stones. The sex distribution of cystine stones is roughly equal.

## Factors affecting crystal formation in urine

**Stasis or the presence of a nucleus,** such as necrotic tissue or bacterial cell wall material, may promote crystal formation, or nucleation, in metastable urine (supersaturated urine, without crystal formation). In some patients, a small calcium stone called a Randall's plaque may form at the tip of a renal papilla. When detached, this can act as a nucleus for stone formation.

**Urine pH** influences the solubility of urinary salts and can vary greatly depending on diet and/or the presence of infection (average pH $\pm$ 6.3). Alkalinization of the urine by urea-splitting bacteria causes precipitation of calcium-magnesium phosphate; acidification below pH 5.5 results in precipitation of uric acid crystals.

**Reduced urine volume** is a critical factor in crystal formation because the saturation concentration of urinary salts is increased, potentially causing a shift from metastable urine to supersaturated urine with crystal formation.

Urine volume (average volume/24 hr, ± 1500 ml) is a function of the volume of fluid consumed, so if small volumes of fluid are consumed, urine volume will be small as well.

**High urinary sodium concentrations** increase urinary calcium levels, with a modest increase in pH. They also decrease urinary citrate concentrations and this, combined with a rise in sodium urate (responsible for nucleation of calcium oxalate), may have a marked influence on urinary stone formation.

### Causes of stone formation

The cause of stone formation is usually only known in a minority of cases (Figure 1.1).

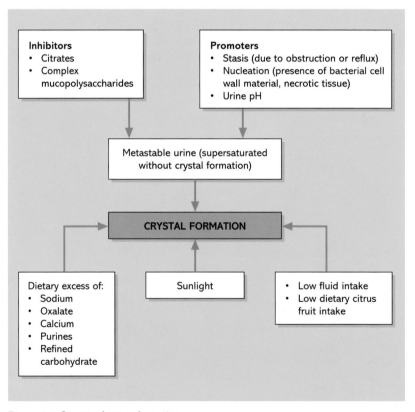

**Figure 1.1** Causes of stone formation.

**Environmental.** The prevalence of urinary stones increases with exposure to sunlight and decreases in a clockwise direction around the world starting in North America. Excessive fluid loss/dehydration, which is often related to occupation, is also considered to be a factor in stone formation.

**Diet.** Excess dietary sodium, oxalate, calcium and purines are associated with an increased rate of stone formation (see Chapter 3). A low fluid intake is also a high risk factor. Insufficient dietary citrus fruit can result in hypocitraturia; conversely a high intake will cause increased potassium citrate excretion and consequently an alkaline load. Urinary oxalate is derived from both metabolic (80%) and dietary sources (20%).

**Hypercalciuria.** Up to 65% of patients with a demonstrable metabolic abnormality have raised calcium excretion due to:
- absorptive hypercalciuria
- renal hypercalciuria
- primary hyperparathyroidism (resorptive).

The biochemical abnormalities in patients with hypercalciuria are listed in Table 1.2.

*Absorptive hypercalciuria* is the most common abnormality and is due to increased intestinal calcium absorption. The high level of calcium in the urine causes calcium oxalate or calcium phosphate crystals to form. The cellular mechanism is unknown, but may or may not be vitamin D dependent. If it is vitamin D dependent, absorptive hypercalciuria can be corrected by a ketoconazole challenge. However, more usually it responds to dietary calcium restriction and sodium cellulose phosphate supplements taken with meals.

*Renal hypercalciuria.* The mechanism is unknown. Pathophysiologically it results in a rise in parathyroid hormone (PTH), which stimulates $1,25\text{-}(OH)_2D$ (vitamin D) production and leads to increased intestinal calcium absorption. The rise in PTH also causes serum phosphate to fall, which is associated with a further rise in $1,25\text{-}(OH)_2D$ production. In patients who have a renal tubular calcium leak, the loss of calcium has a secondary effect on PTH which elevates PTH and maintains normal serum calcium levels to compensate for abnormal renal calcium loss. It may be corrected with thiazide therapy.

TABLE 1.2

**Biochemical abnormalities in patients with hypercalciuria**

**Serum**

| Biochemical abnormality | Calcium | Phosphate | PTH |
|---|---|---|---|
| Absorptive hypercalciuria Type I* | ↑ – | – | ↓ – |
| Absorptive hypercalciuria Type II** | – | – | – |
| Renal hypercalciuria | ↓ – | – | ↑ |
| Primary hyperparathyroidism | ↑ | ↓ | ↑ |

**Urinary calcium**

| Biochemical abnormality | Low calcium diet | Fasting | After 1 g load |
|---|---|---|---|
| Absorptive hypercalciuria Type I* | ↑ | – | ↑ |
| Absorptive hypercalciuria Type II** | – | – | ↑ |
| Renal hypercalciuria | ↑ | ↑ | ↑ |
| Primary hyperparathyroidism | ↑ | ↑ | ↑ |

*Classic primary gut hyperabsorption
**Probably a less severe form of absorptive hypercalciuria Type I
↑, increased; ↓, decreased; –, normal; PTH, parathyroid hormone

*Primary hyperparathyroidism* causes a rise in $1,25\text{-}(OH)_2$ vitamin D with increased intestinal calcium absorption and also increased bone resorption, leading to a higher filtered calcium load. Excess $1,25\text{-}(OH)_2D$ also occurs in up to 50% of patients with sarcoidosis and other granulomatous conditions leading to unregulated $1,25\text{-}(OH)_2D$ production.

**Hyperuricosuria.** Uric acid is an end-product of purine metabolism. Two types of stone can form in hyperuricosuria, depending on urine pH.
- If urine pH is less than 5.5, then primarily uric acid or occasionally calcium oxalate stones form. Uric acid is a weak acid and is only half

ionized at pH 5.75 – if the urine becomes more acidic, most of it is precipitated.

- At a higher pH (> 6.3), calcium oxalate stones tend to form because hyperuricosuria increases the saturation of sodium urate, which induces nucleation of calcium oxalate. Sodium urate may also bind to inactive macromolecules, which act as inhibitors of stone formation.

Hyperuricosuria may also occur if there is a primary metabolic defect, such as in gout or during the excess protein breakdown that occurs during cancer chemotherapy or other catabolic states.

**Hyperoxaluria.** Primary hyperoxaluria is rare and is usually associated with an enzyme (glyoxalate carbogliase or δ-glycerate dehydrogenase) deficiency that results in excess oxalate production. Secondary hyperoxaluria is much more common and is due to increased intestinal oxalate absorption in inflammatory bowel disease or malabsorptive states, such as pancreatic insufficiency. Unabsorbed free fatty acids bind with cations ($Ca^{2+}$, $Mg^{2+}$), thus increasing the pool of unbound, negative oxalate anions for absorption. This effect may be enhanced by increased colonic permeability caused by poorly absorbed bile salts and fatty acids. Bile salts are absorbed by the distal ileum, and resection of this portion of bowel is associated with a doubling of absorption of dietary oxalate. This may be enhanced by an associated alteration of gut flora. The loss of *Oxalobacter formigenes* may result in increased oxalate absorption. Dietary calcium restriction can also result in increased oxalate absorption.

**Cystinuria** is due to an autosomal recessive congenital defect in enzyme transport that causes impaired renal tubular reabsorption of cystine, a product of protein metabolism. As cystine is relatively insoluble, particularly at low urinary pH, this predisposes to stone formation.

**Hypocitraturia.** Citrate potently inhibits aggregation of preformed calcium oxalate crystals and slows heterogeneous nucleation by sodium urate. It binds with urinary calcium, further lowering the availability of free cations. Most patients have idiopathic hypocitraturia, though it is also associated with chronic diarrhoea, inflammatory bowel disease and malabsorption. In these cases, hypocitraturia occurs due to loss of bicarbonate in the stool and the consequent acidosis. In distal renal tubular acidosis, reabsorption of citrate is enhanced, which can also lead to hypocitraturia. In complete renal tubular acidosis, there is an associated fall in bicarbonate. In addition, bone loss due to acidosis leads to hypercalciuria. Other causes of hypocitraturia include the use of thiazide diuretics, due to intracellular acidosis, and urinary infection in which bacteria degrade urinary citrate.

**Recurrent urinary infection** is frequently associated with anatomical abnormalities or scarring that cause either obstruction or ureteric reflux. Urinary tract pathogens encourage struvite stone formation by hydrolysing urea. This leads to the urine becoming alkaline and increased dissociation of phosphate (Figure 1.2). Bacteria can become trapped inside stones, rendering them immune to antibiotic therapy and natural defence mechanisms, and thus these stones can harbour infection and make it impossible to sterilize the urine.

**Other causes** include primary renal disease, chronic bowel inflammation or previous surgery. Obstruction to urine outflow, for example pelviureteric junction obstruction, causes stasis of urine and therefore increases the risk of stone formation. Also, prior stone episodes increase the risk of developing subsequent stones.

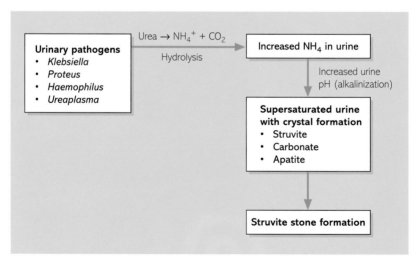

**Figure 1.2** Struvite stone formation.

TABLE 1.3

Inhibitors of stone formation

Low-molecular-weight inhibitors
- Citrate
- Magnesium
- Pyrophosphate

High-molecular-weight inhibitors
- Glycosaminoglycans
- Tamm–Horsfall protein
- Nephrocalcin
- Prothrombin fragment X1

## Inhibitors of stone formation

Two types of substances are present in urine to prevent aggregation of preformed calcium oxalate crystals and slow heterogeneous nucleation by sodium urate (Table 1.3). These include citrate and complex mucopolysaccharides (glycosaminoglycans, GAGs). Presumably the absence/low levels of these substances predispose stone formation in some people. Both inhibitors are reduced in the urine of some stone formers. Low levels of citrate, for example, are often found in stone formers. Administration of citrate often results in cessation of stone formation.

## Key points

- The incidence of stones appears to be increasing
- Stone formation is often multifactorial and complex
- Most stones are due to an underlying metabolic abnormality
- In the majority of patients it is impossible to identify the specific metabolic abnormality responsible for stone formation

## 2 Investigation and diagnosis

Appropriate initial evaluation is essential to establish a firm diagnosis.
Discretion needs to be exercised when deciding which patients require
admission, early intervention and a complex metabolic work-up.

### Presentation

Patients with renal stones may have vague flank pain, or sometimes no
symptoms at all. Often, such stones are discovered incidentally during the
evaluation of unrelated problems. Patients passing ureteric stones often have
severe pain beginning in the flank and radiating around to the groin. Pain
from a stone in the lower ureter may be felt in the testicle or labia and may
cause frequency and urgency of urination. About 85% of ureteric stones
will pass spontaneously. Patients may also present with haematuria,
gastrointestinal upset, irritative voiding symptoms and occasionally with
sepsis if associated with infection or obstruction.

### Assessment and investigations

Patients with a suspected urinary stone should undergo investigation to:
• assess renal anatomy and function
• identify contributing factors
• confirm the diagnosis.
In addition to symptom assessment, a structured history should be taken
(Table 2.1). This is particularly important in recurrent stone formers.
Patients with hyperparathyroidism, certain bowel diseases, or uncontrolled
metabolic abnormalities may form stones at much higher rates. Risk factors
for recurrence are listed in Table 2.2. Results from these investigations will
help to determine optimal treatment and may also identify an underlying
metabolic abnormality.

**Renal anatomy and function.** Today, in most emergency rooms in the
USA the first radiological study obtained in suspected stone patients is a
spiral CT scan. This is much less common in the UK due to a lack
of resources.

TABLE 2.1

**Patient history**

- Occupation
- Any history of stone disease
- Previous treatment
- Family history
- Dietary assessment
- Medical history
  - any history of Crohn's disease, bowel surgery or metabolic disorders
  - drug history
  - sarcoidosis
  - recurrent urinary infection
  - urinary tract surgery, particularly in childhood
  - history of immobilization

TABLE 2.2

**Risk factors for recurrent stone episodes**

- Previous stone disease
- Early age of onset
- Family history
- Associated medical disease
- Metabolic abnormality
- Gender (male)
- Multiple stones

The advantages of spiral CT are:
- radiolucent as well as radiopaque stones are identified
- other intra-abdominal pathology may be identified
- renal anatomy can be assessed.

Disadvantages include the fact that the anatomy of the collecting system is frequently not outlined well enough to plan removal of the stone, and that the patient may still need a urogram or retrograde pyelogram.

*Intravenous urography* should be performed in all patients with
suspected stone disease to assess renal anatomy. In particular, it may
identify:

- anatomical abnormalities, such as horseshoe (abnormal fusion
  of the kidneys at the lower pole) or duplex (separate collecting
  systems within each kidney, upper and lower, each with their
  own ureter)
- caliectasis
- the infundibulo-pelvic angle (see Figure 8.4).

It should be ordered to supplement the spiral CT and should be done if
spiral CT is unavailable.

*Ultrasound* should be used as necessary to assess renal size and scarring
and supplement intravenous urography results.

*Radioisotope diuretic renography* is not performed routinely, but is
helpful if a patient has a history of surgery, staghorn stones or obstruction,
to provide further information about:

- differential renal function
- scarring
- vesico-ureteric reflux.

**First-time stone formers.** It is usually sufficient to assess renal function in
this group by checking:

- for urinary infection
- plasma urea concentration
- plasma creatinine level and electrolytes.

The benefit of detecting metabolic abnormalities of limited significance
must be weighed against the cost and inconvenience of investigation,
particularly as long-term compliance rates for medical therapy are
notoriously low. Serum calcium and uric acid assessment will detect
hypercalcaemia and hyperuricaemia, and this should be the limit of
investigation in this group.

**Recurrent stone formers.** Patients who have had multiple previous stone
episodes, stone surgery or have a history of urinary infection will require
more accurate assessment of renal function, including creatinine clearance
or MAG 3 clearance.

TABLE 2.3

**Normal values of salts**

| | 24-hour urine sample (1.5–2.0 litres) | |
| --- | --- | --- |
| Salt | mmol | mg |
| Sodium | < 200 | 1000–3000 |
| Potassium | 25–125 | 500–1500 |
| Urate | 4–6 | < 600 |
| Oxalate | 5 | < 45 |
| Citrate | 5 | > 320 |
| Phosphate | 50 | 500–1100 |
| Calcium | 7–9 | < 200 |
| | **Serum** | |
| Salt | mmol/litre | mg/100 ml |
| Calcium | 2.10–2.55 | 8.5–10.5 |
| Uric acid | 2.0–3.5 | 2.0–7.0 |
| $K^+$ | 3.6–5.0 | 2.8–4.5 |
| Magnesium | 0.6–1.10 | 1.2 |
| $Na^+$ | 135–145 | 125–138 |
| Bicarbonate | 21–31 | 24–30 |
| Phosphate | 1.5–2.6 | 2.5–4.5 |

**Further investigations.** It is estimated that up to 85% of all stone patients demonstrate some evidence of metabolic abnormality. However, detection of a metabolic abnormality is proportional to the intensity and vigour with which a patient is investigated. A thorough knowledge of the mechanisms of stone formation will help when planning a metabolic work-up and treatment.

For patients with recurrent stones, younger first-time stone formers (including those with a family history of stones), and children, three 24-hour urine samples should be collected to measure urine volume and the parameters shown in Table 2.3. A spot nitroprusside test for cystine should also be performed.

Patients with impaired renal function may need further assessment to exclude renal tubular acidosis and confirm their ability to concentrate urine.

Many patients exhibit features of multiple metabolic abnormalities, such as a high uric acid level, hypercalciuria and elevated sodium excretion. Such patients require careful management and multimodal treatment (see Chapter 3).

## Key points

- Spiral CT has replaced intravenous urography in diagnosis of acute flank pain in the USA
- Assessment should include anatomical, functional and contributing factors
- Screening for metabolic factors should be undertaken in recurrent stone formers, children, younger first-time stone formers and those with a family history

# 3 Management

In the past, renal and ureteric stones were removed by open surgery, not treated, or, in the case of ureteric stones, allowed to pass spontaneously. In the era of non-invasive techniques, such as endourology and shock-wave lithotripsy (SWL), few patients are subjected to open surgery and the indications for treatment have undergone subtle changes. Because of the minimally invasive nature of current techniques, many 'asymptomatic' stones, which would not have been operated on in the past, are now often treated electively. Such treatment may be justified in that it prevents an acute stone event happening at an unpredictable, inconvenient time. About one-third of such stones pass spontaneously, if not treated, but not always without symptoms.

## Prevention

For first-time stone formers, the mainstay of prevention of further stone formation is maintenance of a high fluid intake throughout the day and night after removal of the initial stone. Dietary measures are usually not warranted, though avoidance of excessive consumption of calcium-rich foods seems sensible. However, patients with recurrent stones and no demonstrable metabolic abnormality, may need to adjust their lifestyle and adhere to stricter dietary recommendations.

## Lifestyle changes

**Fluid intake.** Increasing urinary volume is the simplest step in the prevention of recurrent stones. This is the so-called stone clinic effect. Patients should be instructed to increase their fluid intake sufficient to produce a urine volume of 2–2.5 litres/day. This usually means a fluid intake of at least 3 litres/day, assuming average activity. Increased activity means increased sensible and insensible fluid loss, which must be made up by increased fluid intake.

**Diet.** Studies have shown that only 20% of patients continue to follow dietary advice 2 years after first receiving it (Table 3.1).

TABLE 3.1

**Dietary recommendations for stone formers in the absence of a demonstrable metabolic abnormality**

- Minimum fluid intake (2.5 litres/24 hours)
- Low sodium intake (< 3 g/day)
- Moderate restriction of red meat intake
- Limit oxalate-rich foods (see Table 3.3)
- Increase citric fruit intake
- Moderate restriction of dairy produce intake
- Restrict refined sugars
- Increase consumption of oily fish

*Calcium.* Limitation of dietary calcium intake is usually not necessary. Hypercalciuria will not be affected by minor changes in calcium intake and can be more easily managed using thiazide diuretics. Foods vary in calcium content and typical values are shown in Table 3.2.

*Oxalate.* Some patients with high urinary oxalate benefit from extra dietary calcium. Of a 100–1000 mg daily intake of dietary oxalate, only 2–5% is absorbed and excreted. Therefore, because so little oxalate is absorbed, a low oxalate diet is not indicated for routine stone patients, though such a diet may be useful if the patient has hyperoxaluria. Oxalate-rich foods are listed in Table 3.3.

TABLE 3.2

**Calcium-rich foods (values per standard serving)**

- All dairy produce
  - yoghurt (415 mg)
  - milk (396 mg)
  - cheese (204–272 mg)
  - ice cream (236 mg)
- Rhubarb (266 mg)
- Cheese pizza (220 mg)

- Chocolate (70–149 mg)
- Baked beans (133 mg)
- Sardines (107 mg)
- Broccoli (89 mg)
- Herring (49 mg)
- White bread (30 mg)

TABLE 3.3
**Oxalate-rich foods (values per standard serving)**

- Rhubarb (720–1032 mg)
- Spinach (570–675 mg)
- Beetroot (573 mg)
- Cocoa powder (174 mg)
- Okra (117 mg)
- Tea (72 mg)
- Peanuts (52 mg)
- Soft fruits (13–66 mg)

*Protein.* The recommended daily allowance of protein (0.8 g/kg body weight) allows 160–210 g of meat, poultry or fish daily. Most individuals in affluent western societies exceed this amount easily, resulting in uric acid production.

*Sodium.* In western countries, sodium intake is often in excess of 300 mEq/day and may increase calcium excretion considerably. Sodium restriction may be part of the management of hypercalciuria. Restriction to 150 mEq/day has a profound lowering effect on calcium excretion and will reduce the incidence of stone formation. Sources of excess dietary sodium are listed in Table 3.4.

## Medical therapy

**Analgesia.** Passage of a ureteric stone is painful and often requires narcotics. Typically, the pain is episodic requiring multiple trips to the emergency

TABLE 3.4
**Sources of excess dietary sodium (values per standard serving)**

- Salt shaker (100 mmol)
- Fast food (28–110 mmol)
- Processed meats (60 mmol)
- Canned food, such as soups and vegetables (29–52 mmol)

room in search of pain control. Pethidine, diclofenac or meperidine is typically necessary to control symptoms, which have little to do with the size of the stone.

**Diuretics.** Thiazide diuretics are commonly used to decrease urinary calcium levels in recurrent stone formers with hypercalciuria and patients with medullary sponge kidneys and stones. Most such diuretics will elevate serum calcium.

**Potassium citrate or lemon juice** may be prescribed for normo-calciuric patients to increase urinary citrate levels. Citrate is an inhibitor of renal stone formation and this drug is indicated specifically in those patients who are hypocitraturic. Some feel it should be given to any stone former and it has been shown to increase the percentage of stone clearance after shock-wave lithotripsy of renal stones.

**Allopurinol** is a drug that reduces endogenous uric acid production and hence the level of serum uric acid. It will also help reduce the level of urinary uric acid. It is indicated in those patients who form uric acid stones.

**Sodium cellulose phosphate** is used in patients with severe Type I absorptive hypercalciuria, primarily as an alternative to thiazides. It binds with calcium in the gut and limits absorption of calcium.

**Penicillamine** is used in the treatment of cystinuria and cystine stones by decreasing excretion of cystine. It is used primarily as part of the treatment programme for patients whose disease is difficult to manage.

**Antibiotics** are given to treat documented urinary tract infection. While there is no substitute for complete stone removal for patients with infected stones, antibiotic suppressive therapy may help prevent recurrent stone formation and is indicated in those with recurrent urinary tract infections.

**Combination therapy.** Patients with complex metabolic abnormalities require careful management (Table 3.5). For example, patients with a

1,25-$(OH)_2$D excess and hyperuricosuric calcium stone formation may be given a combination of thiazide diuretics, allopurinol and potassium citrate. Together, these agents reduce urinary calcium levels and prevent urate-induced crystallization of calcium salts, by lowering calcium and uric acid excretion and raising urinary pH. It is probably best to manage such patients in specialized metabolic stone units.

**Parathyroidectomy.** About 3% of stone patients have hyperparathyroidism with elevated serum calcium levels. Removal of the parathyroid adenoma will decrease parathormone levels, which will normalize the serum calcium.

## Stone fragmentation and removal
Indications for intervention are listed in Table 3.6.

**Open surgery.** In the modern era, open surgery for urinary stone removal is uncommon, with an overall incidence of no more than approximately 1% of stone patients. In the kidney, surgery may be necessary for stones that cannot be removed by any reasonable number of SWL and/or percutaneous nephrolithotomy (PNL) procedures. Occasionally, a mid-ureteric stone is so fixed or inaccessible that surgery is required. Laparoscopy may be an appropriate alternative to incisional surgery.

**Minimally invasive methods of stone fragmentation and removal** are now commonplace and include:
- ureteroscopy (see Chapter 5)
- percutaneous nephrolithotomy (see Chapter 7)
- shock-wave lithotripsy (see Chapter 8).

Nephrostomy tube placement and/or stent insertion is used to gain access to, and allow drainage from, the kidney and to maintain ureteric patency (see Chapter 6).

## Important factors in renal stone management
Several critical factors determine optimal management of renal stones.

**Size, composition and hardness** are the most important factors. The cross-sectional area of a 2.5 cm diameter stone, the size below which

TABLE 3.5

**Management of patients with complex metabolic abnormalities**

| Abnormality | Cause |
|---|---|
| Low urine volume | Low fluid intake<br>Environmental factors |
| High sodium | Excess dietary sodium |
| High oxalate | Dietary primary oxaluria |
| High calcium | • Absorptive hypercalciuria<br>• Renal leak<br>• Primary hyperparathyroidism |
| High uric acid | • Dietary<br>• Gout<br>• Excess protein breakdown<br>• Chemotherapy |
| Low citrate | Low dietary intake |
| Low urine pH | Gout |
| Cystinuria | Autosomal recessive defect |

most urologists would use SWL, is approximately 495 mm². A comparison of SWL or PNL for treatment of struvite stones showed that when the cross-sectional area of the stone was 500 mm² or less, stone-free rates following each treatment were more or less the same. Above 500 mm², stone-free rates dropped considerably with SWL, indicating that PNL should be used to treat these larger stones. This same rule is likely to apply to non-infected stones.

| Management | Effect |
| --- | --- |
| ↑ Fluid intake | ↓ Saturation of urine with stone-forming salts |
| ↓ Salt intake<br>• Check urea and electrolytes | Restores urinary citrate<br>↓ Sodium urate<br>↓ Urinary calcium<br>↑ Macromolecule activity |
| • Restrict intake of certain foods<br>• Treat cause | ↓ Urinary calcium/oxalate level |
| • Restrict dietary calcium<br>• Sodium cellulose phosphate<br>• Thiazide diuretic<br>• Potassium citrate, lemon juice<br>• Parathyroidectomy | ↓ Calcium excretion<br>↓ Calcium absorption<br>↓ Sodium urate<br>↑ Alkalinization of urine |
| • Restrict all meat intake<br>• Check urine pH<br>• Allopurinol<br>• Potassium citrate | ↓ Sodium urate excretion leading to ↑ macromolecule activity |
| • Lemon juice<br>• Potassium citrate<br>• Citrus fruits | ↑ Citrate level<br>Alkalinization of urine<br>↑ Solubility of calcium salts |
| Potassium citrate | ↑ Citrate level<br>Alkalinization of urine |
| ↑ Fluid intake<br>• Penicillamine<br>• Potassium citrate | ↓ Urinary saturation<br>Alkalinization of urine |

Stone hardness is very difficult to assess radiographically, though the density of an adjacent rib can be used for reference. However, dense, radiopaque stones are unlikely to fragment readily.

**Renal anatomy, presence of obstruction and location.** These factors are interrelated. If the collecting system is obstructed, it is unrealistic to expect stone fragments to pass. This is most common when stones are in a caliceal

TABLE 3.6

**Indications for intervention**

A stone should be fragmented and/or removed if it:

- does not pass after 1 month or causes constant pain
- is too large to pass spontaneously
- obstructs urine flow
- causes chronic urinary tract infection
- damages kidney tissue or causes significant bleeding
- has increased in size

diverticulum (Figure 3.1) or behind an ureteropelvic junction (UPJ) obstruction (Figure 3.2).

## Important factors in ureteric stone management

**Size.** About 85% of ureteric stones pass spontaneously. The chance of spontaneous passage is approximately 85% if the stone is 4 mm in greatest

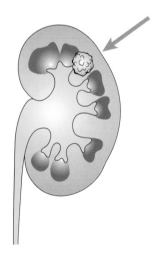

**Figure 3.1** A stone in a caliceal diverticulum. A retrograde or antegrade endoscopic procedure will enable the surgeon to correct the underlying pathology or obstruction.

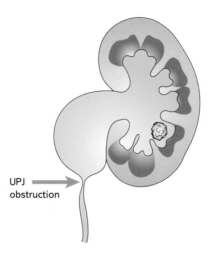

**Figure 3.2** Ureteropelvic junction (UPJ) obstruction contributes to stone formation and prevents fragments from passing. These stones are often calcium oxalate monohydrate (jackstone) stones.

diameter or less, 50% if it is 4–5 mm, and 10% if it is 5 mm or more. Many other factors are also involved. For example, round stones are more likely to pass than irregular-shaped ones and patients who have passed stones of a certain size previously may be expected to do so again. The decision to remove a passable stone may be forced by a patient's intractable pain, multiple trips to the emergency department or unwillingness to wait an unpredictable length of time for spontaneous passage.

**Location.** The position of a stone in the ureter may influence the likelihood of spontaneous passage (upper ureteric stones pass less commonly), however passage is mainly related to stone size. The position of a stone in the ureter will determine the method of fragmentation/removal. In the lower ureter (the portion of the ureter below the iliac vessels), either SWL or ureteroscopy is appropriate for primary treatment, though the preferred technique is the subject of considerable debate and the decision often depends on patient preference (see Tables 5.1 and 8.4).

For most stones in the upper ureter, SWL is the procedure of choice, though the advent of high-quality, small, flexible-steerable ureteroscopes has made ureteroscopy an increasingly reliable alternative. The role of PNL in the upper ureter is usually confined to that of a salvage procedure after failed SWL, but it may be a first choice for certain large, hard stones in the upper ureter or UPJ.

## Key points

- 80% of patients fail to follow dietary advice
- Maintenance of a high fluid intake is probably the most effective preventative treatment
- 85% of ureteric stones still pass spontaneously
- PNL produces higher stone-free rates than SWL for stones > 2.5 cm in diameter
- Scalpel surgery is needed for < 1% of patients with renal stones

# 4 Equipment

Effective management of urinary stones depends on using the correct tools, and to achieve optimum treatment results it is essential to have a clear understanding of treatment technology, its effects on the urinary tract and the patient in general, together with an awareness of potential problems.

## Optical link

The optical link (Figure 4.1) is used to locate and visualize the stone and comprises:

- endoscope
- light source and light-guide cable
- camera and monitor.

**Endoscope.** All rigid endoscopes are based on a rod-lens system, in which images are received at the objective and light is transmitted through a fibre-

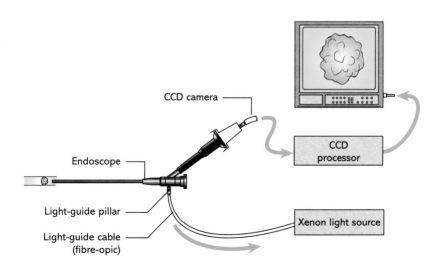

**Figure 4.1** The optical link.

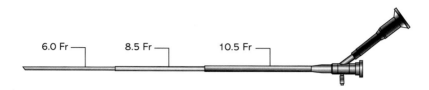

6.0 Fr ———— 8.5 Fr ———— 10.5 Fr ————

**Figure 4.2** A 6.0 Fr rigid ureteroscope is typically 6.0 Fr for several centimetres, after which it increases in size to provide rigidity. Passage of the instrument to the upper ureter will dilate the ureter to 10.5 Fr.

optic bundle. Flexible instruments transmit light and receive images through the same fibre-optic bundle. Rod lenses supply a clear, bright image. While current fibre-optics yield images of excellent quality, there is a slight fuzziness to the image.

*Ureteroscopes* are used for endoscopic examination of the ureteric lumen and renal collecting system. Rigid ureteroscopes are available in sizes from 4.5 to 11.5 Fr (measured at the tip of the instrument; 3 Fr = 1 mm diameter). Most ureteroscopes increase in size towards the eyepiece to provide rigidity to the shaft of the instrument (Figure 4.2). The most commonly used rigid instruments measure 6.0, 7.5 or 8.5 Fr and use fibre optics rather than rod-lens optics. Image quality is excellent and more than adequate for stone management. Flexible-steerable ureteroscopes are now made in sizes 7.5–8.5 Fr with working channels for instruments up to 3.0 Fr. Despite the usefulness of these instruments, durability is still a problem in routine use.

*Nephroscopes* are rigid instruments used only during direct percutaneous renal surgery to view the renal collecting system and extract stones or remove tumours of the collecting system. Most are 28.0 Fr and use rod-lens optics, though some employ fibre optics as part of the eyepiece (Figure 4.3). Recently, smaller instruments (21.0 Fr) have become popular, particularly for use in children. The working channels in these nephroscopes can accommodate instruments up to 11.0 Fr, and stones up to 8 mm in diameter can usually be extracted through the sheaths using forceps or a basket.

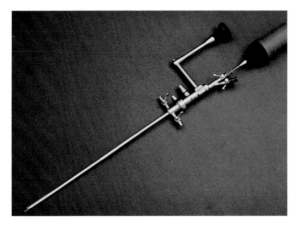

Figure 4.3 A percutaneous nephroscope with a right-angled lens, which allows the operator to view the stone on which the ultrasonic probe is placed.

**Light source and light-guide cable.** Most light sources used in endoscopy rely on powerful xenon or halogen bulbs as high-intensity light is required for optimal transmission of images via the camera. Light is transmitted from the light source to the lens system via a fibre-optic or liquid light-guide cable. The fibre optic in the light-guide cable may become damaged over time resulting in significant light loss. Liquid cables do not suffer from this problem, but are less flexible and significantly more expensive.

**Camera and monitor.** The CCD (charge couple device) camera receives the image from the lens and transmits it to the monitor after processing. Most cameras used routinely in urology contain a single chip, but triple-chip cameras have better image definition and colour transmission, but are heavier and more expensive. The camera can be coupled directly with the lens or via a beam-splitter containing a prism that enables the operator to look directly through the endoscope while the image is transmitted simultaneously to the monitor.

**Image quality.** Potentially, loss of image quality can occur at several sites. It is imperative to check the optical link at the start of each operating list, and a regular maintenance programme will ensure optimal image quality. The major reasons for loss of image quality are listed in Table 4.1. The list is not exhaustive, but demonstrates that attention to detail will optimize image quality and that the majority of problems can be resolved easily by the surgeon or theatre team.

TABLE 4.1

**Reasons for loss of image quality**

| Image | Reason | Action |
|---|---|---|
| None | Incorrect/faulty connections | • Check that power is switched on<br>• Check connections to monitor, camera and light source |
| Blurred | Out of focus | • Correct focus |
| Misty | Water in interface, camera/telescope or camera/beam splitter | • Dry interfaces |
| Glare | Too much light | • Adjust light intensity<br>• Change iris setting<br>• Check correct cable |
| Poor colour reproduction | Incorrect colour balance | • White-balance camera<br>• Monitor settings |

## Stone retrieval devices

Small stones or fragments that can be removed without trauma to the ureter may be retrieved using grasping forceps or one of several types of wire basket (Figure 4.4).

**Grasping forceps** are open-ended, so it is not necessary to pass the instrument beyond the stone. This is particularly useful if oedema is present or for removal of smaller fragments produced by lithotripsy in the presence of an obstructing stone. However, use of these forceps is limited because to grasp the fragment it is necessary to open the jaws of the grasper to an extent that significantly exceeds the diameter of the fragment. Often, this is not possible within the confines of the ureter and sometimes the grasper falls outside the focal range of the ureteroscope. The advantage of forceps is that they allow the operator to release the stone if it is not possible to withdraw it from the ureter easily.

**Baskets.** Choice of basket is a matter for the individual urologist. Confusingly, there are a large number of proprietary baskets available, but

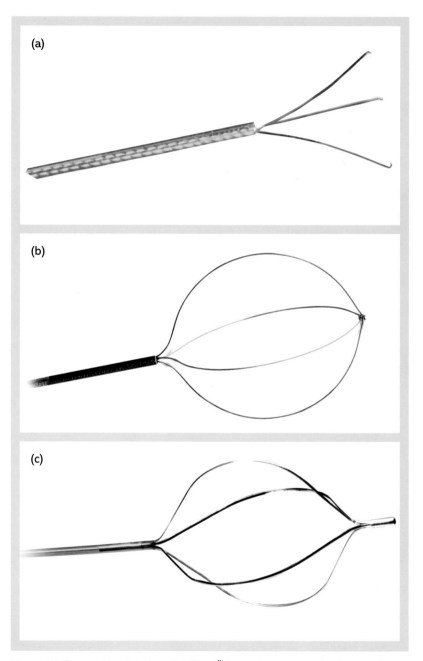

**Figure 4.4** Stone retrieval devices. (a) Tricep™ hooked-prong grasping forceps; (b) Zero Tip™ basket; (c) Segura™ basket.

the basic principles of stone extraction apply to them all. Each consists of an outer sheet of plastic and a braided inner steel wire with a disposable or re-usable opening device at the proximal end to control the basket. Newer baskets are made of nitinol, an alloy with considerable memory properties. All baskets have a minimum of three wires; increasing the number of wires reduces the risk of stone loss during extraction, but may make initial entrapment more difficult.

*Helical baskets* with an end mesh are useful for trawling the ureter to remove small fragments, such as those produced by lithotripsy. However, there is a significant risk of the stone and basket becoming trapped in the ureter and these devices must be used with caution.

*Flat-wire baskets* have greater space between the wires when open. The stone is usually engaged sideways on, allowing easier entrapment and improved control.

*Multiple-fragment retrievers* should be used with extreme caution. It is very easy to 'overfill' the basket while trawling the ureter for fragments resulting in the instrument becoming trapped inside the ureter.

*Tipless baskets* are a new range of nitinol four-wire baskets designed for caliceal stone removal with flexible ureteroscopes. In general, these baskets allow full deflexion of the flexible ureteroscope, and the tipless nature and strength of the basket mean it can be fully deployed in a calix.

## Stents

Ureteric stents are widely used in endourology and successful use much depends on understanding their pathophysiological effect. Stents have two major effects on the ureter:
• cytotoxicity
• paralysis of ureteric function, resulting in ureteric dilatation and/or vesico-ureteric reflux.

The effects on ureteric function appear to be independent of stent size, length or material, though the coating may react with the urothelium and cause inflammation. Stents do not reliably relieve ureteric obstruction and have been reported to produce transient obstruction during the first 24 hours after placement (Figure 4.5). Thus, an *in situ* ureteric stent does not always assure ureteric patency.

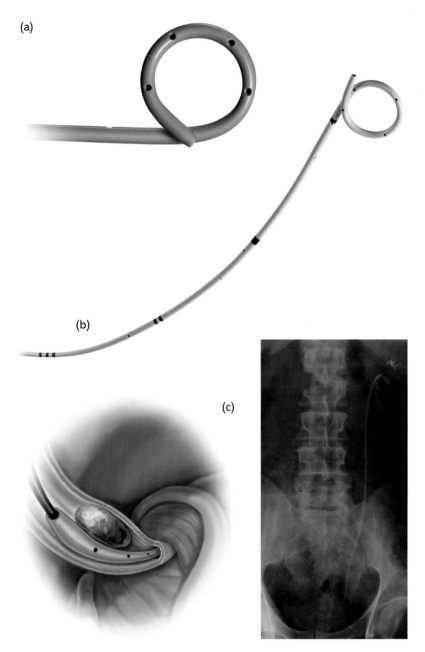

(a)

(b)

(c)

**Figure 4.5** Examples of ureteral stents showing common features: (a) stent tip;
(b) markers at 5 cm intervals (not radio-opaque); (c) tail stent in position.

**Design.** Although stents vary in design, all have common features:
- coils at both ends for retention (pigtail or J)
- calibration in centimetres for accurate placement
- a standard-sized hollow lumen for insertion over a guidewire
- drainage holes throughout the length of the stent.

Recently there have been several changes in design, though there is little evidence that the modifications are an improvement over the original double-pigtail configuration. Most stents are manufactured with a 'dangle' or suture attached to the J-end in the bladder; this allows the patient to remove the stent without visiting their doctor. However, patients must be fully briefed on stent function and given directions about self-removal and appropriate timing for removal. If the dangle is not required, it can be removed during stent placement.

**Materials.** A wide variety of materials have been used in the manufacture of stents. Most stents are made from polyurethane, have differing degrees of rigidity and are available in a variety of lengths and diameters.

A balance is needed between the cytotoxicity of the material and risk of biofilm formation and encrustation (Figure 4.6). Biofilm develops on the surface of indwelling stents and is caused by the adherence of bacterial debris and mucopolysaccharides to the stent surface. It cannot be removed by antibiotic therapy and is associated with an increased risk of encrustation and bacterial colonization.

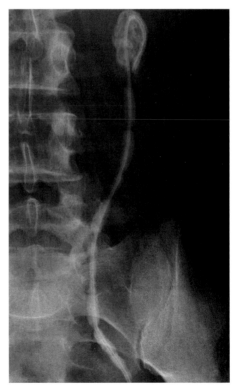

**Figure 4.6** An encrusted stent on plain abdominal radiograph.

The risk of biofilm formation is very variable, but is more common in stone formers than non-stone formers. Stents can be coated with various materials, such as phosphoryl choline (a naturally occurring substance that alters the surface properties of erythrocytes), to reduce the risk of biofilm. Some materials, such as the hydrophilic coating used to ease stent passage, increase the risk of biofilm. Pure silicone stents appear to have the lowest risk of encrustation.

**Sizes.** Stents in sizes 4.8, 6.0, 7.0 and 8.0–8.5 Fr are appropriate for most adult patients, though larger and smaller stents are also available. In most adults, 22 cm and 24 cm stents are of adequate length. However, a particularly tall person may need a 26 cm stent. Special situations may require even longer ones. When a stent is placed antegrade (Figure 4.7), for example as part of an antegrade endopyelotomy, a 26.0 Fr stent is usually

(a)       (b)

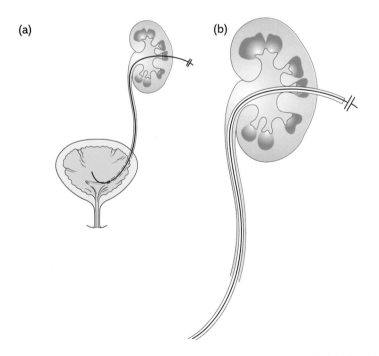

**Figure 4.7** Stents may also be placed using an antegrade approach. (a) First, the radiologist places a guidewire through the flank, down the ureter and into the bladder. (b) The stent is then inserted antegrade over the wire under fluoroscopic control.

necessary to ensure a margin of safety in proper positioning. A specially designed endopyelotomy stent is available, which measures 14.0 Fr in its upper part and 7.0 Fr in its lower portion. However, the authors have not found any advantage in overall success rates with this stent compared with an 8.0 Fr stent. It is also difficult to insert unless the ureter has been previously dilated by stent placement.

In multilength stents, the functional length of the stent varies due to the presence of an extra coil on the distal end, which is straightened out when it is inserted into the ureter. These stents, though attractive in theory, have little additional practical value as the coil tends to reform *in vivo*, changing the position of the stent.

## Percutaneous access and drainage

Dilators. In order to get a nephroscope into the collecting system a track must be created. Usually, these tracks are made by passing dilators, each one larger than the previous one, over a previously placed guidewire. The size to which the track must be dilated depends upon the size of the nephroscope, but is typically 30 Fr. Dilators are passed under fluoroscopic control to ensure that the guidewire does not buckle and that the dilator ends up in the appropriate position.

*Metal aerial telescopic dilators* enable dilatation of the track to a diameter of 30 Fr for percutaneous stone extraction. The inherent rigidity of the dilators makes them particularly useful in patients with perirenal scarring following previous renal surgery, and the system is inexpensive as the dilators are reusable.

*Semi-rigid teflon-coated dilators* (Amplatz) allow variable dilatation of the track, and are disposable and so a relatively expensive option.

*Balloon dilators* allow rapid, one-step dilatation. It is essential that the tip of the balloon is placed within the renal pelvis, otherwise dilatation of the renal parenchyma may not occur. The system contains an Amplatz sheath that slides over the inflated balloon and is relatively easy to operate, though it is not reusable.

Korth fascial knife. This instrument is advanced over a guidewire to a preset depth to gain access when considerable perirenal scarring from previous surgery is present.

**Drainage** is usually achieved postoperatively. A larger-diameter (usually 18–22 Fr) Foley catheter will allow blood and urine to drain, and produce some degree of tamponade of the nephrostomy track. Self-retaining, narrow-diameter (10 Fr), silicone, looped tubes (Cope loop) are widely used for long-term nephrostomy drainage (Figure 4.8).

## Guidewires

These are used to gain and maintain access to the upper urinary tract. They are made of special alloy stainless steel or nitinol wire, and vary in stiffness, diameter and type of tip (Table 4.2). The inner core may be moveable or

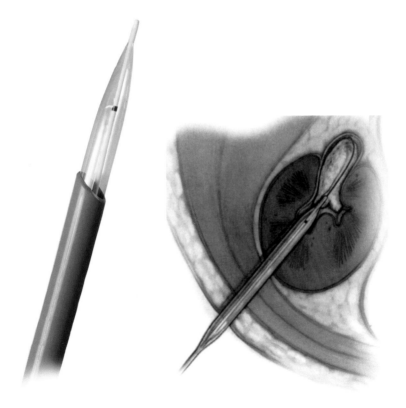

**Figure 4.8** A high-pressure nephrostomy balloon dilatation catheter allows one-step atraumatic dilatation of the nephrostomy track and convenient placement of a working sheath.

TABLE 4.2

**Currently available guidewires**

| | |
|---|---|
| **Diameter (inches)** | 0.025, 0.028, 0.032, 0.035, 0.038 |
| **Length (cm)** | 60–150 |
| **Stiffness** | Standard, stiff, superstiff |
| **Coating** | PTFE, hydrophilic |
| **Colour** | Green, blue, striped, black |
| **Tip design** | Curved, 'J', straight, angled |

TABLE 4.3

**Guidewires suitable for various endourological procedures**

| Indication | Coating | Stiffness | Tip design |
|---|---|---|---|
| Safety wire | PTFE | Standard | Straight |
| Percutaneous access | PTFE | Stiff/superstiff | J |
| Stent insertion | Hydrophilic | Standard/stiff | Straight |
| Flexible ureteroscope insertion | Hydrophilic/PTFE | Standard/stiff | Straight |
| Antegrade stent insertion | PTFE | Stiff/superstiff | Straight |
| Ureteric stricture negotiation/dilatation | Hydrophilic/PTFE | Stiff/superstiff | Angled/straight |

PTFE = polytetrafluoroethylene

fixed and the outer core is coated to reduce friction. The type of coating determines the degree of friction.

A selection of guidewires is necessary for endourological practice because more than one type of wire may be required during a single procedure (Table 4.3). For example, an angled, super-slippery wire may be used to negotiate abnormal ureteric anatomy or bypass a calculus, followed by re-insertion of a co-axial catheter over the wire. This allows replacement with a stiffer, coated wire to facilitate stent insertion during negotiation of a tortuous ureter.

## Extracorporeal stone fragmentation

There are a number of methods of physically fragmenting stones *in situ*. All stone disintegrators, or lithotriptors, consist of the following components:
- shock-wave generator
- focusing system
- coupling mechanism
- localization system.

Currently, four types of lithotriptor are commercially available and there are more than 20 manufacturers worldwide.

**Microexplosives.** An experimental lithotriptor was produced in Japan in the 1980s using lead azide pellets. Shock waves were generated by an underwater explosion and focused with an ellipsoid. The patient was immersed sitting upright in a water bath. Although this method of shock-wave generation is highly efficient, it has not been successful commercially.

**Spark-gap lithotriptors** produce an underwater discharge of a high-voltage electric current that is focused using an ellipsoid reflector (Figure 4.9). The focal pressure may be varied by altering the voltage used to generate the spark discharge.

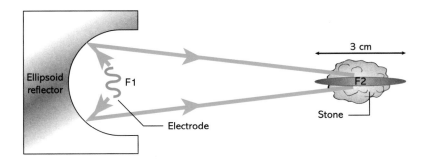

**Figure 4.9** The ellipsoid reflector used in the spark-gap lithotriptor in cross section. F1, shock wave source (spark-gap); F2, second focus at site of stone.

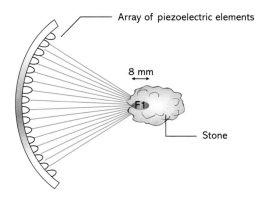

**Figure 4.10** The piezoelectric lithotriptor in cross section. F1, primary focus at site of stone.

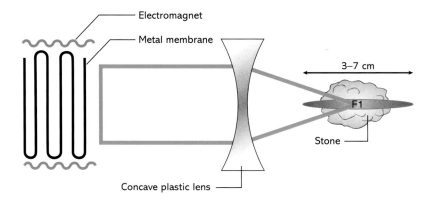

**Figure 4.11** An electromagnetic shock-wave emitter.

**Piezoelectric lithotriptors** involve the simultaneous activation of an array of piezoceramic crystals mounted on a spheroidal dish. A high-voltage electric current is applied, which causes deformity of the crystals and results in a concave shock wave. This converges at the centre of the spheroidal surface on which the crystals are mounted (Figure 4.10).

**Electromagnetic (EMSE) lithotriptors** apply a current to an electromagnetic coil that induces opposing magnetic fields between the coil and an adjacent metallic membrane. The membrane is deflected away from the coil, thus generating a shock wave that travels through water and is focused by means of a biconcave acoustic lens (Figure 4.11).

**Focused laser beam.** Shock waves have been generated using a focused laser beam. However, it has proved too difficult to produce a machine of sufficient commercial reliability because even the smallest particle impurities in the fluid medium deflect the laser beam.

## Intracorporeal stone fragmentation
The various kinds of intracorporeal lithotriptors are compared in Table 4.4.

**Electrohydraulic** lithotriptors work by discharging a high-intensity current at the tip of an electrode. This creates an expanding cavitation bubble that collapses on itself, releasing an acoustic pressure or shock wave. High pressures and heat are produced within a 5 mm zone of the electrode tip, and there is a high risk of ureteric perforation and thus accuracy is important. Smaller diameter electrodes use a lower voltage, which reduces efficacy and may be ineffective for treatment of hard stones.

**Ultrasound.** A longitudinal vibration is induced in a solid metal probe by passage of a high-intensity current into a piezo-ceramic horn. The resulting excitation of the crystals produces an ultrasound wave (20–27 kHz) that

TABLE 4.4

A comparison of intracorporeal stone disintegrators

| Energy source | Cost | Comments |
| --- | --- | --- |
| Electrohydraulic | Inexpensive | Risk of ureteric damage |
| Ultrasound | Moderate | Heat generation |
| Mechanical (pneumatic) | Inexpensive | Propulsion of stone; effective |
| Electrokinetic | Moderate | Less propulsive effect than pneumatic device? |
| Pulsed-dye laser | Expensive | Safe; effective |
| Holmium laser | Expensive | Risk of thermal injury; multipurpose; produces 'dust' |

propels the steel probe to high-frequency sinusoidal vibrations. These vibrations cause the probe to have a 'jackhammer' impact on the stone, which disintegrates at the point of impact. The probe is cooled by continuous irrigation, and debris is evacuated through the hollow lumen using an attached suction pump.

**Mechanical** stone fragmentation uses compressed air (LithoClast®) or a miniature electromagnetic shock-wave emitter (EMSE) device (EKL®, Olympus) to generate a propulsive effect. Fragmentation is proportional to the duration of the energy pulse and amplitude of movement. The subsequent jackhammer impact may result in an unwanted propulsive effect which may cause the stone to migrate proximally up the ureter and into the kidney and thus become inaccessible using the ureteroscope, or the stone may not be able to be sufficiently fragmented; attempts have been made to counteract this effect by applying suction devices to the probe.

Laser

*Pulsed-dye laser.* Laser energy, tuned to a specific wavelength of 520 nm, is transmitted to the stone via a quartz fibre and absorbed. This technique has limited efficacy against cystine and calcium oxalate monohydrate stones because they absorb energy poorly at this wavelength. A localized plasma bubble is produced, which creates a shock wave as it rises and collapses, resulting in an acoustic pressure wave. The dye is biodegradable and may require renewing every few weeks. The dye has a role in the generation of the specific wavelength of the laser.

*Holmium laser.* The holmium:yttrium aluminium garnet (Ho:YAG) laser causes vaporization during direct contact between the fibre and the stone. This solid-state laser transmits energy at 2100 nm via a low water-density quartz fibre 200–1000 µm in diameter. The energy absorbed by the shock wave is produced by expansion and attenuation of a plasma-filled bubble created as the fluid in the focus of the system vaporizes during the laser-induced breakdown. Further transmission of energy occurs through this vapour cavity, the so-called 'Moses' effect. This energy is absorbed by the water component of the stone, leading to thermal disintegration. Approximately 1 joule of energy per pulse (5 Hz) is sufficient to fragment any stone. The very high temperatures at the stone surface may cause thermal damage to the ureter. However, this property can be used to advantage for tissue ablation of transitional cell tumours or benign prostate ablation, making the Ho:YAG laser the only multipurpose laser available for use in urology.

## Irrigation fluid

The choice of irrigation fluid is crucial; generally, normal saline should be used to avoid hypotonic fluid absorption. Low-pressure systems reduce the risk of sepsis, while indiscriminate use of pressure in a closed system, particularly during ureteroscopy, will lead to permanent renal damage, particularly during prolonged procedures or during paediatric endourology.

### Key points

- A thorough working knowledge of the endourological armamentarium will help produce optimum results of stone treatment
- The optical link is complex – minor faults will produce serious loss of image quality
- Nitinol stone baskets represent the state of the art for ease of use and maximum stone retrieval
- Miniaturization of rigid ureteroscopes and the introduction of flexible ureteroscopy has resulted in less ureteric trauma and increased ureteric access
- The Ho:YAG laser and lithoclast operate at opposite extremes of stone fragmentation

## 5  Ureteroscopy

Ureteroscopy is a well-established procedure that is available in most hospitals. The current generation of small, rigid and flexible ureteroscopes has enabled routine endoscopic examination of the entire urinary collecting system; failure to access the area of interest is now rare.

Removal of ureteric stones, particularly from the distal ureter, is the most common indication. Occasionally rigid, but more usually flexible, ureteroscopy is also used for:

- renal stone removal
- diagnostic purposes
- investigation of gross haematuria
- elucidation of filling defects in the collecting system
- investigation of positive urine cytologies
- fulguration of epithelial tumours
- management of ureteric strictures, obstructed calices or UPJ obstruction.

### Technique

Ureteroscopy is often performed as a routine outpatient procedure under general or local anaesthesia. Occasionally, straightforward procedures, particularly in the distal ureter, will require only intravenous sedation.

The surgeon passes the ureteroscope (see Figure 4.2) up the urethra, through the bladder and into the affected ureter. Dilatation of the intramural ureter greatly simplifies the procedure in most patients, permitting easier passage of the ureteroscope and easier removal of stone fragments. However, now that smaller (7.5 Fr) ureteroscopes are available this is done less frequently than previously. A safety guidewire should be placed in all but the simplest cases.

Most stones in the lower ureter can be managed using a rigid ureteroscope (Figure 5.1). The instrument may be passed over a working wire or next to the safety guidewire. In the lower ureter, stones up to approximately 7 mm in size are often extracted using a basket or forceps, particularly if the ureter has been dilated. For stones in the mid- or upper

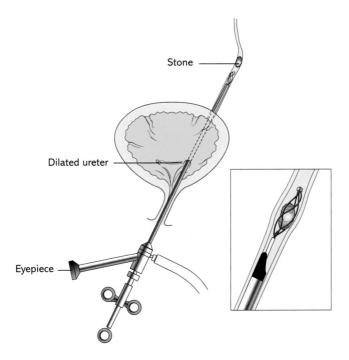

Stone

Dilated ureter

Eyepiece

**Figure 5.1** It is almost always possible to pass the rigid ureteroscope into the lower ureter. The stone can then be extracted with a basket or forceps, or fragmented into pieces using intracorporeal lithotripsy.

ureter, the flexible-steerable ureteroscope is passed over a guidewire until the stone is reached and the wire then removed (Figure 5.2).

Large stones (> 3–4 mm) must be fragmented, using some form of power lithotripsy, into pieces small enough to pass spontaneously or be extracted. Several options are available for intracorporeal stone fragmentation (see Chapter 8). The Ho:YAG laser is preferred because it can fragment any stone in essentially all circumstances. When fragmentation is complete, pieces are either extracted or allowed to pass; spontaneous passage is not always reliable and stone-free rates are higher with routine fragment removal.

Often, a 4.8–6.0 Fr double-pigtail stent (see Chapter 4) is left indwelling for 48 hours or longer after routine ureteroscopy. The stent prevents oedema from obstructing the ureter or colic from the passage of a stone or clot. These advantages are somewhat obviated by the discomfort caused by the stent, but most patients tolerate this if advised of the symptoms, such as dysuria, terminal haematuria and flank discomfort while voiding. If a 'dangle' is used, the patient can remove the stent without visiting their doctor.

In Canada, a prospective, randomized study is currently examining 'stent' versus 'no-stent' after routine ureteroscopy in patients with distal ureteric stones. No patient has undergone balloon dilatation and stones have only been fragmented without extraction. At the time of writing, no difference between the two groups has been reported.

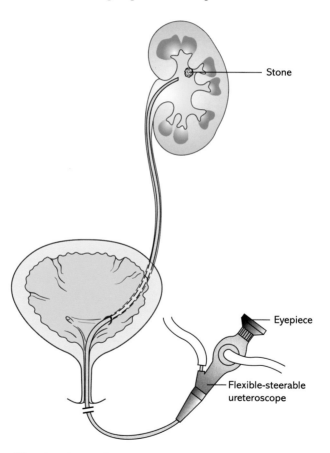

**Figure 5.2** Dilatation of the orifice facilitates introduction of a flexible-steerable ureteroscope. Use of a 7.5 Fr instrument allows evaluation of the entire collecting system.

TABLE 5.1

**Ureteroscopy for primary treatment of ureteric stones**

**Advantages**

- Very high single treatment success rate (essentially 100% if the stone can be visualized)
- Widely available
- Less expensive than SWL

**Disadvantages**

- Invasive
- Requires anaesthesia, though some success under intravenous sedation has been reported

## Results

Ureteroscopy for distal ureteric stone removal is routinely successful, with stone-free rates up to 100% if the stone can be visualized (Table 5.1). In the upper ureter, results are less spectacular, but still excellent in expert hands. Significant complications are uncommon, with a long-term ureteric stricture rate of 0.5%. It is very likely that such strictures after treatment are related to difficult ureteroscopy with injury to the ureteric wall or stone impaction. If the strictures were a function of the particular ureteroscopy method employed, it is likely that such complications would be much more common.

## Key points

- The indications for ureteroscopy are expanding
- Stone-free rates approaching 100% are now commonplace, particularly when a Ho:YAG laser is used

## 6 Nephrostomy tubes and stents

Percutaneous nephrostomy tubes (PNTs) are used to provide:
• permanent or temporary renal drainage
• access to the kidney.

Indications for permanent drainage are uncommon and include patients who are not candidates for an indwelling stent or a surgical procedure to restore ureteric continuity. Temporary PNT placement may be required for urgent or emergency procedures, as well as elective purposes. Emergency indications include temporary drainage required for pain relief or relief of obstruction in the presence of infection. Common situations requiring PNT placement include ureteric obstruction secondary to a stone with accompanying fever or documented infected urine. Relief of obstruction may prevent sepsis and allow definitive stone management on an elective basis. The ureter may be compromised after any surgical procedure, particularly gynaecological surgery, and temporary PNT placement will preserve renal function until the problem can be corrected. Efforts to establish ureteric continuity are often successful with antegrade manipulation through a nephrostomy tract when retrogrades are unsuccessful. Temporary PNT drainage is often necessary after renal surgery, particularly UPJ repair, or as part of percutaneous stone removal. In these circumstances, a PNT can also provide a method of access if necessary.

### Technique

A variety of commercially available nephrostomy kits contain all the equipment necessary for percutaneous access (see Figure 4.8). Percutaneous access is obtained with fluoroscopic or ultrasonic guidance; the former is preferred in the USA whereas the latter is used more commonly in Europe. In skilled hands, differences between these methods are unimportant irrespective of whether they are used for access or percutaneous nephrostomy. The stone is localized preoperatively using ultrasound or intravenous urography. Although the exact point of access depends on patient anatomy, a posterior approach should be avoided if possible, as the

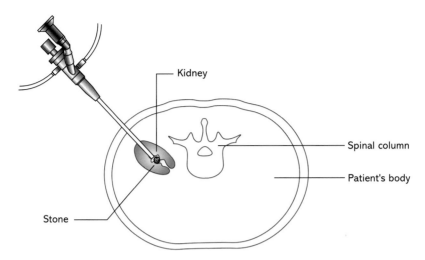

**Figure 6.1** The approach should be as lateral as practical so that the patient does not have to lie on the tube.

patient will have to lie on the tube (Figure 6.1). Entry through a lateral or upper pole calix facilitates working in the ureter, making antegrade stent placement easier. If the indication is drainage alone, it makes little difference where the stent is placed.

Most nephrostomy tubes are self-retaining 10.0–12.0 Fr tubes with a loop in the renal pelvis, created by pulling a suture to curl the end of the tube that lies within the renal collecting system. These tubes should be removed under fluoroscopic control to ensure that the loop is straight and avoid trauma to the kidney. Larger tubes may be placed; however, as access is usually obtained under local anaesthesia with intravenous sedation, it may be prudent to wait before dilating the tract and inserting a larger tube. It is not necessary to sew these tubes to the skin, and chronic antibiotic therapy is not indicated.

## Stents

Double-pigtail indwelling stents (Figure 6.2), also known as 'double-J' stents, are among the most commonly used devices in urology. They are used to maintain ureteric patency in patients with extrinsic ureteric compression due to cancer, or chronic ureteric obstruction resulting from stricture or any other cause. Stents are used to prevent ureteric obstruction

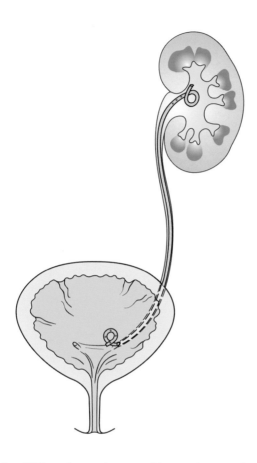

**Figure 6.2** A double-pigtail stent in the correct position. Removal is by cystoscopy under local anaesthetic.

after SWL and sometimes to aid ureteric stone fragmentation during SWL, though there is no evidence to support the latter. Double-pigtail stents are routinely placed after ureteroscopy to prevent ureteric obstruction due to oedema. Stents are also used after either retrograde or antegrade endopyelotomy.

A stent is often placed after a failed endoscopic procedure with a view to re-examination – often a double-pigtail stent will dilate the ureter after several days making endoscopic examination possible.

## Management

Stents may be removed 48–72 hours after routine ureteroscopy. If the stent falls out earlier, it should not be replaced. Longer placement times are needed for traumatic or complicated procedures. Long-term stents should be replaced every 3–6 months to avoid obstruction by debris. Stents that have been 'forgotten' for several years deteriorate and fragment readily. Removing these stents endoscopically often requires both an antegrade and retrograde approach because it is usually impossible to straighten out the J-end for ureteroscopic removal.

## Complications

Despite concerted efforts to design an 'asymptomatic' stent, so far this has not been achieved and every patient who has a stent dislikes it. Patients complain of terminal dysuria, terminal haematuria, and many, particularly men, notice flank pain on voiding because the bladder forces urine up the stent as well as out of the urethra. Bladder symptoms are probably aggravated if a stent is too long. A small stent may become obstructed readily with debris and cause associated symptoms. Although use of the dangle obviates the need for an office visit for stent removal, it increases the risk of unwanted stent removal. This is more common in women who may sit on the dangle while voiding or inadvertently pull the dangle while wiping.

Stents may become calcified, causing problems during removal in patients with active stone disease. This often occurs when a stent is placed during pregnancy. Golf-ball-sized stones can form at the J-ends and the lumen may be totally obstructed by stony material. Fortunately, these stones usually respond to SWL and endoscopic lithotripsy methods.

### Key points

- PNT provides:
    - permanent and temporary renal drainage
    - access to the kidney
- Access can be obtained equally effectively using:
    - fluoroscopy
    - ultrasound guidance

## 7  Percutaneous nephrolithotomy

In 1975, Fernstrom and Johanson created a percutaneous tract directly into the kidney through which a nephroscope could be passed specifically for the purpose of stone removal. Since then, percutaneous nephrolithotomy (PNL) has become a standard procedure for renal stone management. Although in theory PNL is suitable for management of all renal and ureteric stones, in practice it is used mainly for large stones that are unsuitable for SWL and as a salvage procedure for ureteric stones.

### Access

Several factors determine the correct approach to stone management: renal anatomy, stone location and whether the procedure is to serve any other purpose, such as antegrade endopyelotomy. Typically, entry through a middle or lower-pole posterior calix will allow uncomplicated access for a large stone in the renal pelvis. Some prefer an upper-pole caliceal approach and, though this usually allows good access to the collecting system and upper ureter, there is a much higher risk of pleural injury (Figure 7.1). In the USA, most urologists and radiologists use fluoroscopy (see Chapter 6) to access the renal pelvis, whereas ultrasound is preferred in Europe.

Access is readily obtained under local anaesthesia, with intravenous sedation if necessary (Figure 7.2). General anaesthesia is required for tract dilatation and lithotripsy. Usually, the patient is placed prone, but the procedure can be performed with the patient in the flank position.

If a standard sized continuously irrigating 28.0 Fr nephroscope is used, the tract must be dilated to 30.0 Fr to accommodate a 30 Fr Amplatz sheath through which the nephroscope can be placed (Figure 7.3). Alternatively, the nephroscope sheath itself can be used to tamponade the tract (Figure 7.4).

### Technique

The collecting system must be inspected and any clots removed. The stone is evaluated (Figure 7.5) and a decision made about subsequent

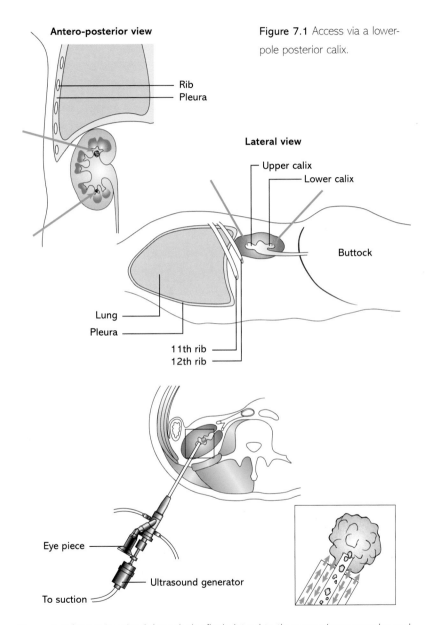

**Figure 7.1** Access via a lower-pole posterior calix.

**Figure 7.2** Access is gained through the flank, lateral to the paraspinous muscles and medial to the colon. The nephroscope is shown at the stone with the ultrasonic probe abutting the stone. As the stone is fragmented, small pieces are aspirated up the probe lumen.

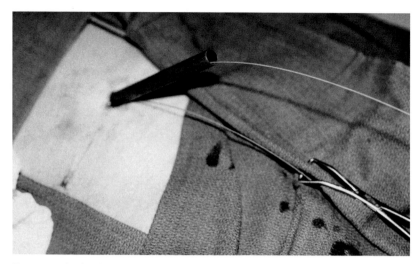

**Figure 7.3** An Amplatz sheath in position through the patient's flank. The safety guidewire is positioned outside the Amplatz sheath, and the working wire is in place through the sheath.

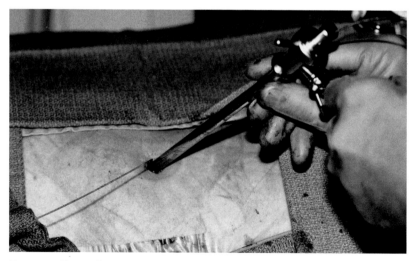

**Figure 7.4** The nephroscope sheath itself, instead of the Amplatz sheath, is used to tamponade the tract.

management. PNL is usually used for large stones and so power lithotripsy is required for stone fragmentation (see Chapter 8). Ultrasound is preferred because pieces can be aspirated up the probe lumen as they are created.

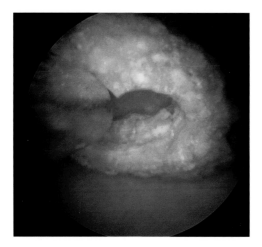

Figure 7.5 The stone is easily visualized with the ultrasonic probe immediately adjacent to it. The hole in the centre has been drilled out by ultrasound.

When the stone has been fragmented and removed, a visual inspection with fluoroscopic assistance will identify any residual stones. If present, they should be removed. A fluoroscopic assessment of the kidney and a plain abdominal radiograph will determine whether the patient is stone-free.

Most, though not all, surgeons leave a 22.0–26.0 Fr nephrostomy tube in place to facilitate re-insertion of the instrument, if necessary. This is a reasonable precaution as PNL is used primarily for difficult problems. Recently, some surgeons have advocated leaving a 8.0–12.0 Fr tube in place to minimize discomfort from the tube, while allowing re-access if needed.

## Complications

**Intrarenal artery damage.** Damage to a branch of an intrarenal artery, either during access or stone removal, is the most significant complication with PNL (overall risk, approximately 0.5%). Patients present with significant gross haematuria, and require transfusion and arteriographic embolization of the bleeding vessel. Knowledge of the intrarenal arterial blood supply can help minimize haemorrhagic complications.

**Venous bleeding,** which is apparent with the irrigation turned down and disappears when irrigation is on, is much more common and usually is obvious during the procedure. Injection of contrast agent into the collecting system often allows identification of the renal vein. Plugging the nephrostomy tube for 30–40 minutes allows the collecting system to tamponade, while concomitantly administering mannitol (or an alternative diuretic) may be very useful in dealing with this problem.

**Extravasation of irrigating fluid** is less likely if the irrigant is allowed to flow around the nephroscope through the Amplatz sheath. Periodically, the total volume of irrigant used should be compared with that collected off the drapes and through the tubes, and any discrepancy noted. If more than approximately 500 ml cannot be accounted for, the surgeon should consider stopping the procedure and continue another day. This may signify that the outstanding volume has been absorbed or extravasated (particularly intravascular extravasation) into the retroperitoneum.

**Adjacent-organ damage.** Occasionally, organs adjacent to the kidney are damaged during access. For example, if the colon is dilated, safe access may be prevented. If the colon is injured, this can usually be managed without the need for open surgery by draining the colon externally with a nephrostomy tube and internally diverting urine using a double-J stent and Foley catheter.

## Results
PNL is strikingly effective, with stone removal rates varying between 95% and 99% in a wide variety of indications. Patients with more complicated conditions, such as complete staghorn calculi or stones associated with difficult access issues, have stone-free rates closer to 80–85%. PNL has the advantages that hospitalization is short (1–3 days) and disability minimal. In addition, if it becomes necessary to stop during the PNL procedure, it can always be continued another day, as long as access remains.

### Key points

- The complication rate is low; those that occur relate to access and nephroscopy
- High stone-free rates can be obtained
- An upper caliceal approach is associated with a higher risk of potential injury

# 8  Shock-wave lithotripsy

Shock-wave lithotripsy involves the application of targeted shock waves, produced externally to the body using a device called a lithotriptor, to fragment stones within the urinary tract. The pieces created pass along the ureter and are voided in the urine via the urethra. In February 1980, the first patient was treated with SWL following years of research collaboration between Dornier and the University of Munich. The Dornier HM-3 was the first lithotriptor to be produced commercially and required general anaesthesia and a water bath in which the patient was suspended by means of a ceiling-mounted gantry. Since then, millions of people have been treated worldwide. Nowadays, the number and types of lithotriptor have grown exponentially (see Chapter 4), and almost all consist of a water-filled cushion placed in contact with skin to provide a coupling mechanism between the lithotriptor and the patient's body. Sedational analgesia is usually sufficient. This is often performed on an outpatient basis, even if a patient requires additional sedation; recovery is immediate.

## Basic principles

Shock waves consist of a single positive pressure front with a steep onset and a gradual decline. Their physical characteristics, peak pressure and energy density differ depending on the mechanism of generation (Figure 8.1). Stones are fragmented by a combination of mechanisms:

- tensile stress
- spalling effect
- cavitation.

Shock waves pass unchanged through water and body tissue until they converge on the focal point, in this instance the stone (Figure 8.2). They are reflected and refracted at acoustical surfaces in the same way as light waves at an optical interface. This is why it is of utmost importance that the lithotriptor cushion is in direct contact with the body with an intervening transducer gel layer. As the shock wave strikes the interface between the stone surface and surrounding urine or renal tissue, a portion is reflected. This creates a *tensile stress* that removes a layer of material from the leading

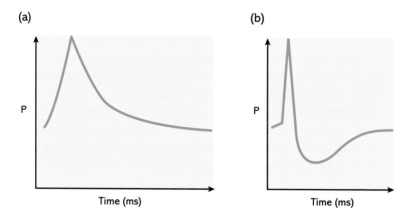

**Figure 8.1** Pressure wave forms produced by (a) the Wolf Piezolith and (b) the Dornier HM-3 lithotriptor.

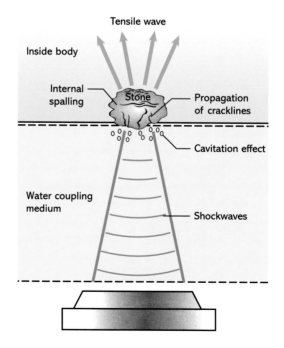

**Figure 8.2** The mechanism of stone fragmentation.

edge of the stone. The bulk of the shock wave passes through the stone and is internally reflected from the back surface, creating a large tensile force that tears a layer of material off the back surface of the stone. The application of multiple shock waves will lead to pulverization of the stone – this is the *spalling effect*.

*Cavitation* bubbles form in a liquid when the tensile force exceeds the forces holding the liquid together. They may contribute to stone fragmentation, as well as causing surrounding tissue damage. Powerful microjets form in bubbles adjacent to the stone surface, producing pressures of up to 225 MPa, and these jets are sufficiently powerful to produce holes in aluminium foil or dent brass plates.

The number of shock waves needed to fragment a stone depends on:
- stone hardness/composition (Table 8.1)
- focal pressure
- energy density
- fluid interface.

The size of fragments produced by lithotripsy varies with the energy of the shock wave. To produce smaller particles, lower energy is required, so a greater number of shock waves are needed to fragment the stone completely. Reasons for lithotripsy failure are shown in Table 8.2.

## Shock-wave lithotripsy as first-line treatment

The decision to use SWL as primary treatment is determined by:

TABLE 8.1

**Stone composition and ease of fragmentation with SWL**

Stones that fragment readily:
- calcium oxalate dihydrate
- uric acid
- struvite

Stones that fragment with difficulty:
- calcium oxalate monohydrate
- cystine
- brushite (calcium phosphate)

TABLE 8.2

**Reasons for lithotripsy failure**

The stone does not fragment because of:

- inaccurate localization
- inadequate power
- lack of expansion chamber
- excessive hardness

Stone fragments do not pass because of:

- large size
- inadequate drainage

- stone size
- stone position
- anatomical features (including obstruction).

The ureter is effectively a conduit that conducts stone fragments from the kidney to the bladder. If the ureter becomes obstructed due to large or numerous fragments, then a steinstrasse will develop (Figure 8.3). Prior stenting of the ureter will increase its capacity and assist passage of fragments; peristaltic ureteric function may be restored by relieving obstruction using a nephrostomy.

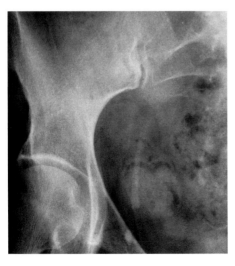

**Figure 8.3** A plain abdominal radiograph showing a blocked ureter with a steinstrasse.

## Choice of localization

The advantages and disadvantages of two methods of stone localization, fluoroscopy and ultrasound (see Chapter 6), are shown in Table 8.3.

## Renal stones

Although SWL may fragment stones in the renal diverticulum or behind a UPJ obstruction and relieve symptoms, it will not treat the underlying pathological problem. It is well known that the stone-free rate after SWL for lower-pole stones is about half that for stones in upper-pole calices. Recently, it has been discovered that the angle the lower-pole infundibulum makes with the renal pelvis has a bearing on the likelihood of stone passage (Figure 8.4). If the angle is less than 70°, spontaneous passage is less likely.

SWL is likely to be less effective for renal stones if:
- a stone is large
- the stone is composed of cystine or 100% calcium oxalate monohydrate
- a stone coexists with obstruction
- the patient's anatomy precludes SWL, e.g. patients with morbid obesity so that the stone cannot be manoeuvred into the focal point
- a stone-free state is important.

TABLE 8.3

**Choice of localization method**

| Method | Advantages | Disadvantages |
|---|---|---|
| Fluoroscopy | • Easy technique<br>• Enables full imaging of the ureter | • Radiation dose<br>• Real-time imaging impossible for duration of treatment |
| Ultrasound | • No radiation<br>• Real-time monitoring of fragmentation<br>• Imaging of radiolucent stones<br>• Small stones more easily visualized | • More difficult technique<br>• Imaging of the mid-ureter impossible |

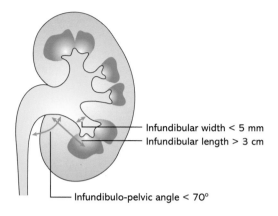

**Figure 8.4** Adverse factors affecting stone clearance after SWL.

Infundibular width < 5 mm
Infundibular length > 3 cm
Infundibulo-pelvic angle < 70°

## Ureteric stones

The advantages and disadvantages of SWL for ureteric stone fragmentation are shown in Table 8.4.

## Analgesia

Three factors affect the ability to give SWL treatment without the need for analgesia:

- the size of the skin aperture (pressure density)
- the size of the shock-wave envelope
- the energy density within the shock wave (focal pressure).

## Tissue damage

Shock waves generated underwater are spherical and must be focused to avoid damage to adjacent tissues. They are focused geometrically by an ellipsoid reflector, or in the case of EMSE by an acoustic lens. The size of the focal volume is a geometric function of the focusing system, and the degree of damage to surrounding soft tissues is related to its size as well as to the focal pressure. The Dornier HM-3 lithotriptor and Siemens Lithostar produced focused shock waves that had significantly larger volumes than those produced by current third-generation machines.

TABLE 8.4

**Shock-wave lithotripsy for primary treatment of ureteric stones**

**Advantages**

- Non-invasive
- Easily repeatable
- Local anaesthesia or intravenous sedation

**Disadvantages**

- High repeat treatment rate
- High ancillary treatment rate
- Later-generation machines are not as effective as original Dornier HM-3
- More expensive in some healthcare systems
- Not routinely available

## Complications

Haematuria is a direct result of shock-wave trauma. Infection may be caused either by bacteria that are liberated during SWL or obstruction caused by stone fragments.

## Key points

- Stones are fragmented by a combination of:
  - cavitation
  - spalling effect
  - tensile stress
- Stones are localized by ultrasound or fluoroscopy
- Lithotripsy for larger stones increases the risk of:
  - residual stone fragments
  - steinstrasse
- The anatomical appearance of the kidney is likely to have an effect on stone clearance

# 9 Guidelines and consensus terminology

Guidelines are preformed practice policies, in any area of medicine, that can be used by physicians as a guide when selecting treatment options for a given disease or condition. The American Urological Association (AUA) began to create guidelines for selected urological topics about 10 years ago. Rather than an 'implicit' approach dependent on expert opinion alone, they chose the reference-based 'explicit' approach pioneered by Eddy *et al*. Relevant literature is reviewed and abstracted, and data combined and meta-analysed. When a guideline document relies on expert opinion, this is stated explicitly.

Treatment recommendations are graded into three levels, depending on the strength of the data supporting the recommendation (Table 9.1). The AUA created guidelines for stones in two areas: staghorn stones were chosen because treatment was controversial and ureteric stones because of their high prevalence and difference of opinion concerning appropriate treatment.

TABLE 9.1

**Treatment recommendations**

**A standard**

Treatment outcomes are sufficiently well known that there is essential unanimity of opinion about what should be done.
This is the most rigid recommendation

**A guideline**

More flexible than a standard; most, but not all, of those who express an opinion agree on the particular intervention

**An option**

There is insufficient evidence to select one option over another.
This is the most flexible recommendation

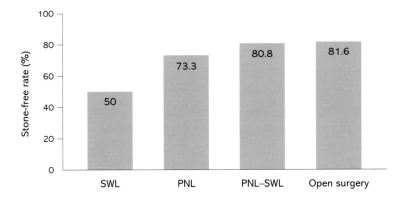

**Figure 9.1** Stone-free rates using different treatment approaches.

## Staghorn stones

Stone-free data were extracted from the peer-reviewed English-language literature on four different treatment approaches:

• SWL alone

• PNL alone

• PNL in combination with SWL or ureteroscopy

• open surgery.

From these data, it is clear that the best results are achieved with combined therapy or open surgery, and that SWL alone is not very effective (Figure 9.1). Furthermore, SWL results in a significantly higher unplanned secondary procedure rate (Table 9.2).

The recommendations of the AUA Clinical Guidelines Panel are summarized in Table 9.3.

## Ureteric stones

The same approach was used for ureteric stones. A MedLine search (1966 to January 1996) yielded 1698 articles, 526 of which were abstracted. Acceptable outcome data were obtained from 327 of these papers. The stone-free data on which guidelines were based are shown in Table 9.4.

Stone treatment results reported in the literature vary enormously, particularly when results are expressed as a function of stone size; there is no consensus on the size of a 'clinically insignificant residual fragment'.

TABLE 9.2

**Primary and secondary procedures and complication rates in the management of staghorn stones***

| Treatment approach | Primary procedures (n) | Secondary procedures (%) | Complication rates (%) |
|---|---|---|---|
| SWL | 2.1 | 42 | 31 |
| PNL | 1.5 | 4.7 | 7.4 |
| Combination (SWL–PNL) | 2.8 | 3.4 | 24.4 |
| Open surgery | 1.0 | 0.2 | 1.2 |

*Adapted from Segura *et al.* 1994

TABLE 9.3

**AUA Guideline Panel recommendations for staghorn stones**

**Standards**

- A newly diagnosed struvite staghorn stone is an indication for active treatment

- The patient must be informed about the four alternatives available for treatment

**Guidelines**

- Percutaneous stone removal, followed by SWL and/or repeat PNL as necessary, should be used for most patients with staghorn stones

- SWL monotherapy is not appropriate for first-line treatment

- Open surgery is not appropriate for first-line treatment

**Options**

- SWL monotherapy and PNL alone are equally effective for certain small volume stones in patients with normal or near-normal anatomy

- Open surgery is appropriate in those patients whose stones cannot be expected to be removed by any reasonable number of SWLs and/or PNLs

- Nephrectomy may be appropriate in some poorly functioning, stone-bearing kidneys

Until recently, most ureteroscopy series reflected the writer's learning curve rather than the results it is possible to achieve with reasonable experience.

TABLE 9.4

**Overall stone-free rates using shock-wave lithotripsy, ureteroscopy or open surgery***

| Treatment approach | Proximal ureter (%) | Distal ureter (%) |
|---|---|---|
| SWL | 83 | 85 |
| Ureteroscopy | 72 | 90 |
| Open surgery | 97 | 87 |

*Adapted from Segura *et al.* 1997

For the purposes of guideline development, the ureter was divided at the iliac vessels into upper and lower portions, and stones were classified as 1 cm or less, or more than 1 cm in size. The following treatment alternatives were considered:
- ureteroscopy
- SWL
- PNL
- open surgery
- 'blind basketing' (basket extraction without fluoroscopy or a safety guidewire).

The Ureteral Stones AUA Clinical Guidelines Panel recommendations are summarized below and in Table 9.5.

**Standards.** Patients must be informed of available treatment modalities, together with their associated risks and benefits.

**Guidelines.** Up to 98% of stones smaller than 0.5 cm in diameter are expected to pass spontaneously, particularly in the distal ureter, and so observation was recommended as initial treatment. The panel also recognized that the time to stone passage, degree of pain, number of trips to the emergency room and other factors all contribute to the decision to intervene.

Stent insertion to increase the efficacy of SWL was not recommended, because no data were found to support this practice, though routine stenting may be justified for other reasons.

Despite limitations, these reference-based guidelines reflect accepted practice reported in the international literature and, therefore, are less likely to contain biased opinion than recommendations developed from expert opinion alone.

International application of these guidelines depends on availability of technology, the particular healthcare system and, possibly, cultural factors.

## Consensus terminology

The efficacy of modern minimally invasive stone management techniques is agreed, but optimal treatment of different stones remains a matter of

TABLE 9.5

**The AUA Clinical Guidelines Panel recommendations for ureteric stones**

| Stone size and position | Standards | Guidelines |
|---|---|---|
| *Proximal ureter* | | |
| ≤ 1 cm | • Open surgery should not be first-line treatment | • SWL is recommended as first-line treatment. If SWL fails or is inappropriate, ureteroscopy or PNL are indicated |
| > 1 cm | • Open surgery should not be first-line treatment | • SWL, PNL and ureteroscopy are all acceptable options |
| *Distal ureter* | | |
| ≤ 1 cm | • Open surgery should not be first-line treatment | • Blind basketing cannot be encouraged as an acceptable treatment choice. SWL and ureteroscopy are both acceptable options |
| > 1 cm | • Blind basketing is not recommended | • Open surgery should not be first-line treatment, though it may be appropriate for certain large stones or in unusual circumstances. SWL and ureteroscopy are both acceptable options |

considerable debate. The literature, at best, is confused and often misleading due to a lack of consensus on the exact meaning of words and phrases used to assess treatment outcome. Also, imprecise definitions are sometimes used to describe primary treatment.

In 1989, representatives from each lithotriptor centre in the UK attended a consensus meeting in Edinburgh to discuss standardization of terms used in lithotriptor treatment and reporting of results. This was reported in the *British Journal of Urology* in 1991 and subsequently discussed and agreed at the 12th World Congress on Endourology in St. Louis in 1994.

In an age where cost-effectiveness and outcomes are closely scrutinized, it is vital that results are reported accurately and in a clear, unambiguous manner. The most commonly used terms with a consensus of their meaning are listed below.

**The lithotriptor.** Reports concerning lithotripsy should include details of the type of machine used in the study, the energy source and the mode of localization.

**Type of generator.** In addition to information about the energy source, the report should contain details of:
- the range of kV used during treatment or the power-intensity setting
- the manufacturer's estimate of peak pressure produced at the focus
- actual pressures delivered by the machine, where possible
- frequency of shock-wave generation, irrespective of whether frequency of generation is constant, or electrocardiographic- (based on the ST segment of the ECG tracing) or respiratory-gating is used.

**Focus.** A statement of the dimensions of the focus should be included.

**Imaging.** Targeting of the stone is currently performed using ultrasound or X-ray; the modality used should be indicated. Some machines can combine ultrasound and fluoroscopy and, if this is the case, the report should specify which modality was used primarily.

**SWL monotherapy.** This term is ambiguous and its use is not recommended. 'SWL' should be used only for treatments that do not require any ancillary procedures; if for example, a stent is inserted as an additional procedure, this should be categorized as 'SWL plus stent insertion'. Similarly, all other elective ancillary procedures, such as preliminary debulking for manipulation of ureteric stones, should be stated and the proportion of patients treated in this way clearly indicated. If the term 'monotherapy' is used, it should be defined unequivocally in the introduction to the paper.

**A session** is defined as a period c$^f$ lithotripsy treatment, the end-point of which is when the patient leaves the machine. Reports should indicate the number (mean and maximum) of shocks given in any one session. Multiple sessions may be given as a course of treatment, the duration of which should be stated.

**Stone.** Reports should state the site, size and type of stone, and the percentage of single and multiple stones. Measurement of single stones should be at the maximum diameter, with the mean and range noted. Stones should be grouped in sizes less than 1.0, 1.0–1.9, 2.0–2.9 or more than 3.0 cm in diameter, and the number of stones in each group stated. For multiple stones, the number of stones and the assessment of 'stone burden' (the summation of maximum diameters) should be stated.

Anatomical or pathological abnormalities, such as medullary sponge kidney or drainage problems, should be stated. Radioisotope renography is desirable, but not essential, for patients with staghorn stones to assess renal function. It is difficult to quantify the stone burden, which should be subdivided into partial and complete, in these patients. However, the number of calices involved should be noted.

**Failure of fragmentation.** The number of cases in which fragmentation has failed and the time at which this was assessed should be recorded.

**Treatment objectives.** It is important that these are defined before results are assessed. For lithotripsy, the main objective is to clear the treated kidney and ureter of all radiological evidence of stones. However, in some instances, the objective may be simply clearance of the targeted stone or symptom relief. If applied, treatment objectives should be stated.

**End of treatment.** Today, lithotripsy may consist of either single or multiple treatment sessions carried out at intervals, ranging from daily to several weeks. Thus, a course of treatment may extend for some time before it is judged to be complete. The end of a treatment course is difficult to define and varies considerably in time. In most cases, treatment ends when the stone has been adequately fragmented and follow up begins.

A further treatment session for residual fragments, 6 months after concluding the initial course of treatment, should be regarded as secondary SWL and constitutes an additional treatment session. However, the number of secondary or 'stir-up' sessions should be clearly identified.

**Stone free** is defined as the absence of calcific opacities in the treated upper urinary tract, the absence of filling defects on IVU, or absence of stone fragments on ultrasound in the case of a non-opaque stone. Examination of a good quality, plain abdominal radiograph is normally sufficient to confirm the absence of stone fragments. Plain nephrotomography may be indicated if it is difficult to visualize the kidney or stone fragments, but it is not recommended as routine assessment for all radiopaque stones treated by lithotripsy. Similarly, IVU, ultrasound and radioisotope diuretic renography may be used in certain cases, particularly those with non-opaque stones, or to assess renal anatomy and function and help determine whether the upper urinary tract is stone free.

**Residual fragments.** There is, as yet, no consensus on the size of fragment that is significant in terms of later recurrence, stone growth, persistence of infection or further symptoms.

## Key points

- Advice to patients regarding treatment should be evidence-based
- Use of agreed terminology will facilitate the development of acceptable standards, guidelines and options

## 10 / Future trends

Evidence-based management of urinary stones, together with technical advances, will determine future treatment trends. These will be influenced further by the advent of managed care with cash limits for management of a stone episode. Recognition that endourological skills can be taught and practised in the skills laboratory using artificial, yet realistic, models will improve skills and widen the horizons of those practising endourology.

Specific areas of importance are listed in Table 10.1 and discussed below.

### Flexible ureteroscopy

Smaller-diameter instruments (7.5 Fr) with full 180° movement in both directions at the distal tip are now available for routine use. These instruments have never been easier to use, and the larger instrument channel combined with superior optics will result in expanding indications for flexible ureteroscopy and rapid uptake of the technique by all endourologists. Reliability remains a problem, but better training will improve the longevity of these endoscopes. Instrument and device

TABLE 10.1

Future trends in urinary stone management

- Greater surgical intervention
  - flexible ureteroscopy
  - increased use of PNL
  - use of mini-perc
- More critical use of SWL
  - fewer re-treatments
  - better pre-treatment assessment
- Biodegradable ureteric stents
- Improved instrumentation
- Increased use of day-case surgery

manufacturers are responding to the challenge, and producing baskets and graspers that allow retrieval of stones in any part of the collecting system.

The Ho:YAG laser is firmly established as a safe and effective means of stone fragmentation, and the emerging role of this laser in the treatment of urothelial tumours and the prostate makes this tool a far more economical option than previously. Its use, combined with small-diameter ureteroscopes, will make day-case treatment of quite complex stones a feasible option.

## Increased role for PNL

Managed care and limited reimbursement for a single-stone episode will focus the urologist's attention on efficient, as well as least-invasive, methods of stone clearance. Evidence from the Lower Pole Study Group in the USA suggests that the least-invasive treatment (SWL) is not necessarily the most effective for stone clearance. At least one manufacturer has recognized this, and used balloon technology to enable easier establishment of the nephrostomy track. Other innovative ideas will almost certainly follow and make this technically challenging procedure available to all urologists who manage stones.

The advent of the mini-perc technique, which uses a smaller diameter (16 Fr) percutaneous tract into the kidney and a smaller Fr nephroscope, is interesting and reduces the trauma of percutaneous access. However, it has yet to find full acceptance among endourologists. Instrument technology currently used in minimal-access surgery may lead to further advances in this area.

## Ureteric stents

Two major drawbacks for patients are stent discomfort and the need for a further procedure to remove the stent. Novel stent designs with changes to the retaining lower pigtail, which causes bladder irritation and stent miniaturization, may yet reduce stent-related problems. Continuing work in the field of biodegradable stents may result in a stent that can be custom-fitted and manufactured to degrade at a predetermined time after insertion.

## Shock-wave lithotripsy

Changes in the use of SWL are inevitable in view of work suggesting that stone clearance is influenced by caliceal anatomy. Published reports are conflicting, but further studies are underway. Together with the fact that stone size is an important predictor of outcome and complications, this finding must surely result in more-critical case selection. This will also be influenced by more-objective predictors of outcome, such as neural networks that utilize large completed databases and are able to recognize trends and thus predict the success of treatment given many variables. Such networks have proved capable of predicting outcome more successfully than standard statistics.

## Training in endourology

Increased pressure on time and the high cost of occupying an operating theatre must surely influence teaching and assessment of technical skills. There is compelling evidence in the surgical literature to indicate that the skills of endourology, endoperception, endocoordination, endodexterity and endotouch can all be improved with practice. The 20% or so of surgeons who will never possess these skills can also be identified readily by psychomotor testing using computer models. Realistic skills models are being developed to facilitate training in endourology, including percutaneous access.

Political and economic changes that will affect care cannot be predicted with confidence, but there seems little doubt that the management of stone disease in the 21st century must have both a scientific basis and a sound economic rationale. The lack of ability to carry out a procedure or the mere availability of an item of equipment will no longer be sufficient grounds to recommend treatment. Adherence to guidelines and precise use of terminology to define outcome will become a necessary feature in the daily life of the endourologist who wishes to manage stone disease.

## Key points

- New technology will expand the indications for ureteroscopy and PNL
- Biodegradable stents and new stent designs may reduce the high incidence of stent-related problems
- Training is the key to reducing the learning curve of the novice endourologist

# Key references

## AETIOLOGY, INVESTIGATION AND DIAGNOSIS

Coe FL, Favus MJ, Pak CYC et al. Kidney Stones Medical and Surgical Management. Philadelphia, New York: Lippincott-Raven, 1996:1109.

Nordin BEC, Need AG, Morris HA. Metabolic Bone and Stone Disease. 3rd edn. Edinburgh, London, Madrid, Melbourne, New York, Tokyo: Churchill Livingstone, 1993:492.

Resnick MI. New trends in medical evaluation and treatment of patients with urolithiasis. Br J Urol 1991;67:398.

## URETEROSCOPY

Devarjan R, Ashraf M, Beck RO et al. Holmium:YAG lasertripsy for ureteric calculi: an experience of 300 procedures. Br J Urol 1998;82:342–7.

Harmon WJ, Sershon PD, Blute ML et al. Ureteroscopy: current practice and long-term complications. J Urol 1997;157: 28–32.

Turk TM, Jenkins AD. A comparison of ureteroscopy to in situ extracorporeal shock-wave lithotripsy for the treatment of distal ureteral calculi. J Urol 1999;161:45–6.

## NEPHROSTOMY TUBES AND STENTS

Keane PF, Bonner MC, Johnstone SR et al. Characterisation of biofilm and encrustation on ureteric stents in vivo. Br J Urol 1974;73:687–91.

Ryan PC, Lennon GM, Maclean PA, Fitzpatrick JM. The effects of acute and chronic JJ stent placement on upper urinary tract mobility and calculus transit. Br J Urol 1994;74: 434–9.

## PERCUTANEOUS NEPHROLITHOTOMY

Lingeman JE, Coury TA, Newman DM et al. Comparison of results and morbidity of percutaneous nephrostolithotomy and extracorporeal shock wave lithotripsy. J Urol 1987;138:485–90.

Segura JW, Patterson DE, LeRoy AJ et al. Percutaneous removal of kidney stones: review of 1,000 cases. J Urol 1985;134: 1077–81.

## LITHOTRIPSY

Chaussy CG, Schmiedt E, Jocham D et al. First clinical experience with extracorporeally induced destruction of kidney stones by shock waves. J Urol 1981;127:417–20.

Dretler SP. An evaluation of ureteral laser lithotripsy: 225 consecutive patients. J Urol 1990;143:267–71.

Elbahannasy AM, Shalhav AL, Hoenig DM et al. Lower caliceal stone clearance after shock wave lithotripsy or ureteroscopy: the impact of lower pole radiographic anatomy. J Urol 1998;159: 676–82.

Grasso M, Bagley DH. Endoscopic pulsed-dye laser lithotripsy: 159 consecutive cases. J Endourol 1994;8:25–7.

Gravenstein JS, Peter K. *Extracorporeal Shock-Wave Lithotripsy for Renal Stone Disease.* Boston: Butterworths, 1985.

Keeley FX, Pillai M, Smith G *et al.* Electrokinetic lithotripsy: safety efficacy and limitations of a new form of ballistic lithotripsy. *Br J Urol* 1999;84:261–3.

Lam HS, Lingeman JE, Russo R, Chua GT. Stone surface area determination techniques: a unifying concept of staghorn stone burden assessment. *J Urol* 1992;148:1026–9.

Marberger M. Disintegration of renal and ureteric calculi with ultrasound. *Urol Clin North Am* 1983;10:729–36.

Moussa SA, Keeley FX Jr, Smith G *et al.* Clearance of lower pole stones following SWL: the effect of infundibulo-pelvic angle. *J Urol* 1998;159(Suppl):Abstract 122.

Naqvi SAA, Khaliq M, Zafar MN, Rizvi SAH. Treatment of ureteric stones. Comparison of laser and pneumatic lithotripsy. *Br J Urol* 1994;74:694–8.

Teichman JM, Vassar GJ, Glickman RD *et al.* Holmium:YAG lithotripsy: photothermal mechanism converts uric acid calculi to cyanide. *J Urol* 1998;160:320–4.

Teichman JMH, Vassar GJ, Bishoff JTR *et al.* Holmium YAG lithotripsy yields smaller fragments than lithoclast, pulsed dye laser or electrohydraulic lithotripsy. *J Urol* 1998;159:17–23.

Wilscher MK, Conway JM, Babayan RK. Safety and efficacy of electrohydraulic lithotripsy by ureteroscopy. *J Urol* 1988;140:957–8.

## GUIDELINES AND CONSENSUS TERMINOLOGY

Segura JW, Preminger GM, Assimos DG *et al.* Ureteral Stones Clinical Guidelines Panel summary report on the management of ureteral calculi. The American Urological Association. *J Urol* 1997;158: 1919–21.

Segura JW, Preminger GM, Assimos DG *et al.* Nephrolithiasis Clinical Guidelines Panel summary report on the management of staghorn calculi. The American Urological Association Nephrolithiasis Clinical Guidelines Panel. *J Urol* 1994; 151:1648–51.

Tolley DA, Wallace DM, Tiptaft R. First consensus conference on lithotriptor terminology. *Br J Urol* 1991;67:9–12.

# Index

acidification 7
acidosis 12, 18
aetiology 6–13
alkalinization 7, 12, 24
allopurinol 22, 23, 24
American Urological Association (AUA) see guidelines
analgesia 21–2
antibiotics 22
apatite 12
baskets 4, 30, 32–4, 45, 46, 47, 69, 70, 75
bicarbonate 12, 17
bile salts 11
bone resorption 10, 12
calcium 4, 9–10, 11, 16, 20, 23, 24
    salts 6, 7, 8, 9, 17
    see also oxalate; phosphates
caliectasis 4, 16
caliceal diverticulum 26
carbohydrates, refined 6, 8, 20
carbonates 12
case selection 76
chemotherapy 11, 23
citrates 8, 11–12, 13, 17, 22, 23, 24
citrus fruit 8, 9, 20, 24
colonic permeability 11
combination therapy 22–4
compliance rates 16
computerized tomography see CT
consensus terminology 70–3
creatinine 16
Crohn's disease 15
crystal formation 4, 6, 7–8
    see also nucleation
CT 6–7, 14–15, 16, 18
cystine 6, 7, 17, 61, 63
cystinuria 11, 22, 23
cystoscopy 52
dairy produce 20
day-case surgery 74, 75
dehydration 9
diagnosis see investigation and diagnosis

diarrhoea 11
diet and urinary stones 6, 9, 15, 19–21, 23, 28
    recommendations 20–1
dilatation 38, 39, 40, 48, 54
diuretics 12, 22
    see also thiazide
dysuria 48, 53
economics of healthcare 5, 76
endoscopes 4, 5, 29–30
endoscopy 26, 53
    image quality 31–2, 45
endourology 45, 71, 74, 75
    training 76
entrapping 4
    see also basket; equipment; forceps
equipment 29–45, 46–8, 50–2
    improved 74
extracorporeal stone fragmentation 5
    equipment 41–3
family history 15, 17, 18
filling defects see IVU
first-time stone formers 6, 15, 16, 18
flexible ureteroscopy 74–5
fluid intake 8, 9, 19, 20, 23, 24, 28
fluoroscopy 4, 50, 51, 53, 54, 57, 63, 65, 69, 71
forceps 30, 32, 46, 47
frequency 14
future trends 74–6
gastrointestinal upset 14
gender differences 6, 7, 15
geographical location and urinary stones 6
gout 11, 23
guidelines 66–70, 76
guidewires 38, 39–41, 46, 56, 69
haematuria 14, 46, 48, 53, 57, 65
history-taking 14, 15
hydronephrosis 4, 6
hypercalciuria 9–10, 12, 18, 20, 21, 22, 23

absorptive 9, 10
    biochemical abnormalities 10
    renal 9, 10
hyperoxaluria 11, 20
hyperparathyroidism, primary 9, 10, 23
hyperuricaemia 16
hyperuricosuria 10–11, 23
hypocitraturia 11–12, 22
infection 6, 7, 8, 50, 65, 73
inflammatory bowel disease 11, 12
infundibulo-pelvic angle 16, 63, 64
intracorporeal stone fragmentation 5, 47
    equipment 43–5
intravenous urography see IVU
investigation and diagnosis 14–18, 46
irrigation fluid 45, 57–8
irritation on voiding 14
IVU 4, 16, 18, 50, 73
jackstone 4, 27
ketoconazole 9
kidney damage 6
laparoscopy 23
lasers 43, 44–5, 47, 49, 75
    expanding use for 75
lithotripsy see SWL
lithotriptors see SWL
localization of stones see fluoroscopy; ultrasound
MAG 3 16
magnesium 7, 13, 17
malabsorption 11
management 19–28, 52–3, 54
medical therapy 21–4
metabolic abnormality see metabolism
metabolism 9, 11, 13, 14, 15, 16, 17, 18
    managing abnormality 22–4
metastable urine 4, 7, 8
mini-perc technique 74, 75
mucopolysaccharides 8, 12, 36
nephrectomy 68

nephrolithotomy *see* PNL
nephroscopes 4, 30–1, 54, 55, 56, 75
nephrostomy 4, 39, 62
  complications 53
  management 52–3
  technique 50–1
  *see also* tubes and stents
nephrotomography 73
nucleation 4, 7, 8, 11
obstruction 6, 8, 12, 14, 16, 26, 27, 34, 46, 50, 51, 53, 62, 65
optical link 29–2, 45
outcome prediction 76
oxalate 4, 7, 8, 9, 10, 11, 17, 23, 24, 61, 63
  in foods 20, 21
*Oxalobacter formigenes* 11
paediatric endourology 45
pain 14, 18, 53
  relief 21–2, 50
pancreatic insufficiency 11
parathyroid hormone *see* PTH
parathyroidectomy 4, 23
pelviureteric junction *see* UPJ
penicillamine 22, 24
percutaneous nephrolithotomy *see* PNL
percutaneous nephrostomy tubes (PNTs) *see* tubes and stents
pH 7, 8, 10–11, 23
  *see also* acidification; alkalinization
phosphates 7, 9, 10, 17, 61
PNL 4, 23, 24, 28, 54–8, 67, 68, 70, 74, 75, 76
  access 54, 55
  complications 57–8
  equipment 38–9
  results 58
  technique 54–7
potassium 9, 17
prevalence 6
prevention 19
protein, animal 6, 20, 21, 23
PTH 4, 9, 10
purines 8, 9, 10
radioisotope renography 4, 16, 72, 73
radiolucent stones 7, 15, 63, 73
radiopaque stone 15, 73

Randall's plaque 7
recurrence 6, 12, 14, 15, 16, 73
reflux 8, 12, 16, 34
renal anatomy 14, 15, 16, 18, 25, 54, 65, 72, 73
renal collecting system 4, 5, 30, 51
renal stones 46
  management 25–6, 28, 54
  SWL 63
renography *see* radioisotope renography
retrograde pyelogram 15
risk factors 9, 14, 15
salts, normal values of 17
sarcoidosis 10, 15
scarring 16, 38
sepsis 14, 50
shock-wave lithotripsy *see* SWL
sodium 8, 9, 17, 18, 20, 21, 23, 24
staghorn stones 4, 5, 16, 58, 66, 67, 68, 72
stasis 7, 8, 12
steinstrasse 4, 62, 65
stents *see* tubes and stents
stone formation 6
  causes 8–12
  inhibitors 13
stone fragmentation and removal 23–6, 75
  *see also* extracorporeal; intracorporeal; SWL
stone retrieval devices *see* equipment
struvite 4, 6, 7, 12, 61, 68
sunlight 8, 9
supersaturated urine 4, 7, 8
  *see also* metastable urine
surgery
  as cause 12, 15
  as treatment 23, 28, 67, 68, 69, 70
  *see also* PNL and other invasive procedures
surgical stones 6
SWL 4, 5, 19, 22, 23, 24, 27, 28, 49, 53, 54, 59–65, 67, 68, 69, 70, 71–2, 73, 74, 75–6
  analgesia 59, 64
  basic principles 59–61

complications 65
  failure 62
  tissue damage 64
  symptom assessment 14, 74
  technical skill identification 76
  terminology *see* consensus terminology
  thiazide 9, 12, 20, 23, 24
  *see also* diuretics
  training 76
  treatment recommendations 66
tubes and stents 4, 23, 34–8, 40, 47–8, 50–3, 69, 75
  biodegradable stents 74, 75, 76
  cytotoxicity of material 34, 36–7
ultrasound 16, 43–4, 50, 53, 54, 56, 57, 63, 65, 71, 73
UPJ 4, 12, 26, 27, 28, 46, 50, 63
urates 6, 11, 12, 17, 24
urea 16, 24
ureteric stones 14, 46, 49, 66, 67–69
  location 27–8
  management 26–8, 54
  SWL 64, 65
ureteropelvic junction *see* UPJ
ureterorenoscopy 5
ureteroscopes 4, 5, 27, 30, 40, 45, 74, 75
  *see also* ureteroscopy
ureteroscopy 5, 23, 24, 27, 45, 46–9, 52, 67, 69, 70, 74–5, 76
  advantages/disadvantages 49
  results 49
  technique 46–8
urgency 14
uric acid 7, 10–11, 16, 18, 21, 22, 23, 61
urinary collecting system 6, 15, 26, 46, 75
urinary pathogens 12
urinary tract infection 4, 6, 16, 25
  recurrent 12, 15, 22
urine volume 7–8, 19
urogram 15
vitamin D 9